STUDY GUIDE
TO ACCOMPANY

ADULT
HEALTH
NURSING

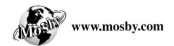 www.mosby.com

STUDY GUIDE

TO ACCOMPANY

ADULT HEALTH NURSING

THIRD EDITION

BRENDA GOODNER, RN, MSN, PhD, CS
Psychiatric Clinical Specialist
Director, Pain Management Program
Rio Grande Health Center, Inc.
El Paso, Texas

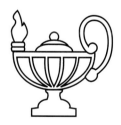

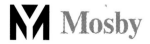

St. Louis Baltimore Boston Carlsbad Chicago Minneapolis New York Philadelphia Portland
London Milan Sydney Tokyo Toronto

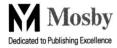
Mosby
Dedicated to Publishing Excellence

Publisher Sally Schrefer
Editors Yvonne Alexopoulos/Susan R. Epstein
Associate Developmental Editor Kimberly A. Netterville
Project Manager Gayle May Morris
Associate Production Editor Lisa M. Kearney
Designer Amy Buxton
Manufacturing Manager Betty Mueller

THIRD EDITION

Composition by Black Dot Group
Printing/binding by Plus Communications

Mosby, Inc.
11830 Westline Industrial Drive
St. Louis, Missouri 63146

International Standard Book Number
0-323-00153-X

99 00 01 02 03/9 8 7 6 5 4 3 2 1

PREFACE

study guide is designed to accompany the third
ion of Christensen and Kockrow's *Adult Health
sing* to assist students in focusing their study skills
he important content presented in the text.

V FEATURES AND ORGANIZATION

new edition has been thoroughly reviewed and
fully revised to ensure accuracy. A new
emporary and visually attractive design has been
rporated to provide a student-friendly learning
ronment. The following study aids are included
ach chapter to facilitate student comprehension
learning:

apter Summary recaps and highlights important
ntent in the corresponding chapter in text.

arning Objectives reflect those in the text, so that
rning in both books is clearly delineated and not
gmented.

y Terms and Definitions in new matching
rmat help students to measure their success in
istering key concepts.

inforcing Key Points help students to focus on
portant concepts presented in the text. Page
mbers are found in the answer key for quick
erence to the text.

plication of Clinical Skills help students to
actice skills and reinforce knowledge that is

mostly required in real-life clinical situations.
Information needed to accomplish these skills is
detailed in the text.

- *New* Exercises in Fundamental Concepts presented
  in fill-in-the blank format review the fundamental
  material discussed in the corresponding chapter in
  the text.
- Exercises in Critical Thinking presented in writing
  and discussion format help promote clinical
  decision-making abilities.
- Multiple-choice Study Questions are provided to
  help students evaluate learning while becoming
  familiar with the type of questions they will
  encounter during testing.

ACKNOWLEDGMENTS

I would like to thank the staff at Mosby for the
opportunity to write this new edition, and for expert
guidance and assistance in preparation of the
manuscript. Their patience and assistance were
invaluable. I would also like to express my
appreciation to Barbara Christensen and Elaine
Kockrow for writing an excellent textbook on which
to base the information in this study guide. The
content is well organized and it was a pleasure to
work with the level of educational material offered.

Brenda Goodner

CONTENTS

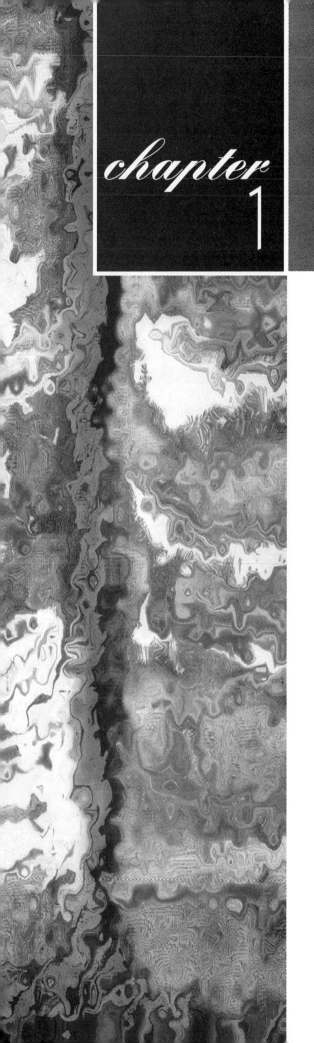

chapter 1

Introduction to Anatomy and Physiology

CHAPTER SUMMARY

Chapter 1 focuses on the anatomy and physiology of the human body. The three imaginary body planes are described, and the body cavities are detailed. The abdominal region is divided and detailed according to its four regions, and the abdominopelvic region is divided into nine regions. The structures of the cell are dissected and labeled, including the process of cellular function and reproduction. The complex functioning of tissues and organs is presented, with details on the four major types of tissue; and, finally, the nine major systems of the body are recognized along with their specific functions.

LEARNING OBJECTIVES

After reading the chapter in the textbook and working through the chapter in this study guide, the student should be able to do the following:

- Define the key terms found in the matching exercises.
- Use each word of a given list of anatomical terminology in a sentence.
- Define the difference between anatomy and physiology.
- Demonstrate an understanding of the body planes by labeling a diagram appropriately.
- Identify and define three major components of the cell.
- Describe the function of adenosine triphosphate (ATP).
- Discuss the stages of mitosis, and explain the importance of cellular reproduction.

- Differentiate among tissues, organs, and systems.
- Describe the four types of tissues.
- Discuss the two types of epithelial membranes.
- List the body systems and the organs contained in each system, and give an example of their functions.
- Differentiate between active and passive transport processes that act to move substances through cell membranes.

KEY TERMS AND DEFINITIONS

_____ 1. Active transport
_____ 2. Anatomy
_____ 3. Cytoplasm
_____ 4. Dorsal
_____ 5. Effusion
_____ 6. Homeostasis
_____ 7. Membrane
_____ 8. Mitosis
_____ 9. Nucleus
_____ 10. Organ
_____ 11. Osmosis
_____ 12. Passive transport
_____ 13. Phagocytosis
_____ 14. Physiology
_____ 15. Pinocytosis
_____ 16. System
_____ 17. Tissue
_____ 18. Ventral

a. The movement of small molecules across the membrane of a cell by diffusion
b. Composed largely of a gel-like substance that contains water, food, minerals, enzymes, and other specialized materials
c. An organization of varying numbers and kinds of organs arranged so that they can together perform complex functions for the body
d. A group of several different kinds of tissues arranged so that they can together perform a common function
e. Explains the function of various structures and how they interrelate to one another
f. Thin sheets of tissue that serve many functions in the body
g. To face forward; the front of the body
h. Type of cell division in which each daughter cell contains the same number of chromosomes as the parent cells
i. Permits a cell to engulf or to surround any foreign material and to digest it
j. Toward the back

k. An organization of many similar cells that act together to perform a common function
l. The study, classification, and description of structures and organs of the body
m. The process by which extracellular fluid is taken into the cell
n. The movement of materials across the membrane of a cell by means of chemical activity that allows the cell to admit larger molecules than would otherwise be able to enter
o. The largest organelle within the cell; it is responsible for cell reproduction and control of the other organelles
p. The passage of water across a semipermeable membrane, with the water molecules going from the less concentrated solution to the more concentrated solution
q. A relative constancy in the internal environment of the body, naturally maintained by adaptive responses that promote healthy survival
r. The escape of fluid from anatomical vessels

REINFORCING KEY POINTS

1. Define and differentiate between the anatomy and physiology of the human body.

2. Discuss the anatomical terms regarding positioning of the body.

3. Describe how the body is divided into three imaginary planes, and name them.

4. Discuss what it means to say a cell is "selectively permeable."

5. Define deoxyribonucleic acid (DNA) and ribonucleic acid (RNA), and in the process explain why DNA is called the "chemical blueprint" and RNA is called the "chemical messenger."

6. Explain what the spindle-shaped rods are that carry the genes that are responsible for an organism's traits.

7. Describe what happens to the cell during the four stages of mitosis.

8. Discuss the importance and function of epithelial tissue.

9. Describe the process of active transport.

10. Describe the process of passive transport.

11. Name the three important functions the epithelial tissue serves.

12. Identify each type of muscle shown below:

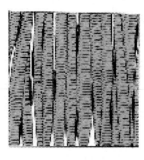 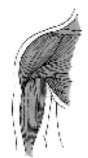

_____

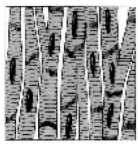 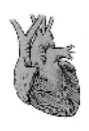

_____

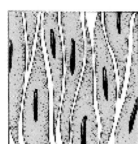 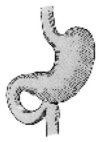

_____

APPLICATION OF CLINICAL SKILLS

1. Perform a head-to-toe systems assessment of the nine body systems, and describe the body functions of each system.

2. Analyze how the body systems compensate to maintain homeostasis.

3. In assessing a patient, divide the abdominal region into nine regions and discuss the assessment of each region.

EXERCISES IN FUNDAMENTAL CONCEPTS

1. In anatomical terminology, posterior means
   _____ .

2. The term *lateral* means _____ .

3. The protein factories inside the cell are
   _____ .

4. The substance that contains the genetic code, or
   blueprint, of the body is _____ .

5. Cell division actually begins to take place during
   the following stage of mitosis, which is called
   _____ .

6. Each body cell in humans contains _____ chromosomes, and chromosomes exist and work in
   _____ .

7. The study, classification, and description of
   structures and organs of the body are known as
   _____ .

8. The process and function of the body, its structures, and how they interrelate with one another
   are known as _____ .

9. The tissue that is primarily responsible for the
   protection of the body is _____ .

10. The word used to describe a part of the body
    nearest the origin of the structure or nearest the
    trunk is _____ .

11. The _____ plane of the body runs
    lengthwise from the front to the back.

12. The _____ cavity contains the
    heart, blood vessels, and lungs; whereas the
    _____ cavity contains the liver,
    gallbladder, stomach, pancreas, and intestines.

EXERCISES IN CRITICAL THINKING

Topics for Writing

1. Sketch the typical cell structure, and review the
   functions of each component that makes up a
   cell.

2. List and describe the phases the cell goes
   through during mitosis.

Topics for Discussion

1. Discuss the structural organization of the body,
   beginning with the atom and working through
   the systems of the body.

2. Discuss how the four major types of tissue within
   the body compose the organs.

3. Discuss the functions of the nine major systems
   in the body.

4. Discuss the difference between active transport
   and passive transport, giving examples of each.

5. Discuss the process of phagocytosis.

STUDY QUESTIONS

1. The nurse is preparing to assess the large intestine of Mr. Parker, who is undergoing a regular
   physical examination. The large intestine is
   found in the body region known as the:
   a. Epigastric
   b. Right iliac
   c. Left hypochondriac
   d. Right hypochondriac

2. Biofeedback is for a patient who is having a lot
   of stress. Biofeedback is used to exert control on:
   a. Nervous tissue
   b. Striated tissue
   c. Visceral muscle
   d. Dendrites and axons

3. During a physical examination the nurse will assess the liver in the:
   a. Right upper quadrant
   b. Left upper quadrant
   c. Right lower quadrant
   d. Left lower quadrant

4. During peritoneal dialysis, small solutes diffuse from blood vessels, but blood proteins do not diffuse. This transport process is called:
   a. Active
   b. Passive
   c. Simple
   d. Osmosis

5. In performing an assessment the nurse is aware that the thick, slippery material that protects parts of the body from bacterial invasion is (are) called:
   a. Visceral cells
   b. Connective tissue
   c. Nonstriated cells
   d. Mucous membranes

6. The process in which solid particles in a fluid move from an area of higher concentration to an area of lower concentration is called:
   a. Diffusion
   b. Osmosis
   c. Filtration
   d. Hypertonicity

7. When a cell engulfs or surrounds foreign material, this process is called:
   a. Diffusion
   b. Absorption
   c. Pinocytosis
   d. Phagocytosis

8. Neurons are nerve cells that have three parts. Their function is to:
   a. Transmit impulses
   b. Support and nourish cells
   c. Exert involuntary control
   d. Enhance voluntary controls

9. It is important for the nurse to know that cardiac tissue is striated, involuntary tissue that branches out to form networks found only in the wall of the heart. This type of tissue is:
   a. Muscle
   b. Nervous
   c. Epithelial
   d. Connective

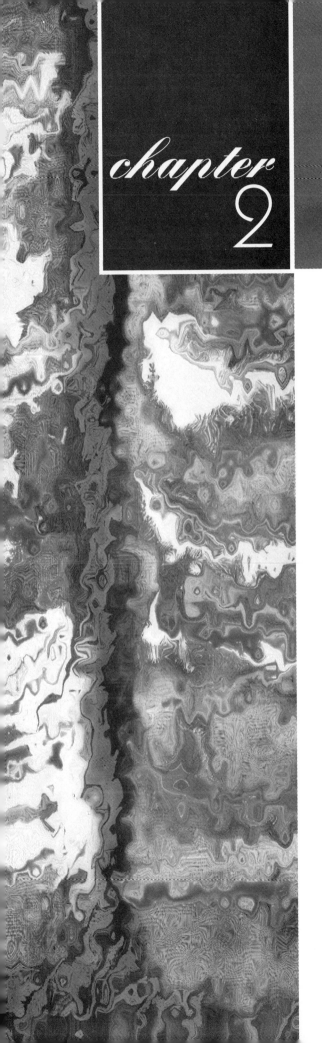

chapter 2

Care of the Patient with an Immune Disorder

CHAPTER SUMMARY

Chapter 2 describes the nature of immunity, including the two major types of immunity and how the mechanisms of the immune response protect people from disease. How the body responds with different types of immunity is detailed. The complement system is explained. Hypersensitivity conditions, such as urticaria, hay fever, and dermatitis, are discussed, in addition to extensive discussion of the medical management of these disorders. Details regarding medications are included. The aggressive treatment of anaphylaxis is discussed, including a comprehensive nursing care plan. An explanation of immunodeficiency is presented, as are transfusion and transplant reactions.

LEARNING OBJECTIVES

After reading the chapter in the textbook and working through the chapter in this study guide, the student should be able to do the following:

- Define key terms found in the matching exercises.
- Differentiate between natural and acquired immunity.
- Review the mechanisms of immune response.
- Compare and contrast humoral and cell-mediated immunity.
- Explain the concepts of immunocompetency, immunodeficiency, and autoimmunity.

- Discuss five factors that influence the development of hypersensitivity.
- Identify the clinical manifestations of anaphylaxis.
- Discuss selection of blood donors, type and cross-matching, and storage and administration protocol of blood in the prevention of a transfusion reaction.
- Outline the immediate aggressive treatment of anaphylaxis.
- Discuss the causation of autoimmune disorders.
- Explain an immunodeficiency disease.

KEY TERMS AND DEFINITIONS

———————— 1. Adaptive immunity
———————— 2. Allergen
———————— 3. Antigen
———————— 4. Attenuated
———————— 5. Autoimmune
———————— 6. Autologous
———————— 7. Cellular immunity
———————— 8. Humoral immunity
———————— 9. Hypersensitivity
———————— 10. Immunocompetent
———————— 11. Immunodeficiency
———————— 12. Immunology
———————— 13. Immunosuppressive
———————— 14. Innate immunity

a. An abnormal condition of the immune system in which cellular or humoral immunity is inadequate and resistance to infection is decreased
b. Pertaining to a tissue occurring naturally and derived from the same individual
c. The body's first line of defense; provides physical and chemical barriers to invading pathogens and protects against the external environment
d. A substance that can produce a hypersensitive reaction in the body but is not necessarily harmful
e. The mechanism of acquired immunity characterized by the dominant role of small T cells
f. Provides a specific reaction to each invading antigen and has the unique ability to remember the antigen that caused the attack
g. The study of the immune system
h. An inappropriate and excessive response of the immune system to a sensitizing antigen
i. A substance recognized by the body as foreign that can trigger an immune response
j. The administration of agents that significantly interfere with the ability of the immune system to respond to antigenic stimulation by inhibiting cellular and humoral immunity
k. The process of weakening the degree of virulence of a disease organism
l. Pertaining to the development of an immune response (autoantibodies or cellular immune response) to one's own tissues
m. The ability of an immune system to mobilize and deploy its antibodies and other responses to stimulation by an antigen
n. One of the two forms of immunity that respond to antigens, such as bacteria and foreign tissue

REINFORCING KEY POINTS

1. List the three main functions of the immune system.

2. Discuss the body's first line of defense, and name this kind of immunity.

3. Discuss the body's second line of defense, and name this kind of immunity.

4. Define specific immunity, and differentiate it from nonspecific immunity.

5. Discuss how the cells of the immune system (macrophages and lymphocytes) function to protect the body.

6. Describe what happens when an infectious agent enters the body.

7. Describe where the B cells and T cells originate in the body.

8. Discuss how lymphokine is produced and its significance.

9. Explain the function of T cells and how and under what conditions they provide immunity.

10. Explain the function of B cells and how and under what conditions they proliferate and provide immunity.

11. Describe the role of antigens in providing immunity.

12. Discuss the concept of humoral immunity and how it is mediated.

13. Describe the complement system and how it works.

14. Discuss how cellular immunity is stimulated and what it is effective against.

15. Explain what it means to say a vaccine is attenuated.

16. Define and differentiate the following immune response disorders:
    a. Autoimmunity

    b. Hypersensitivity

    c. Immunodeficiency

17. Discuss five factors that influence hypersensitivity.

18. Review the organization of the immune system by labeling the figure below:

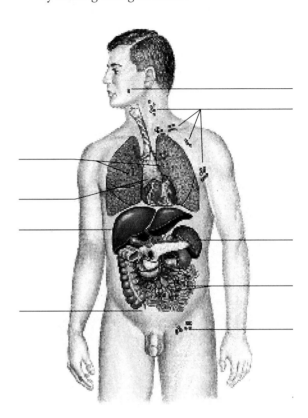

APPLICATION OF CLINICAL SKILLS

1. Explain the diagnostic test involved in a hypersensitivity illness.

2. Write a patient teaching plan for the patient with allergic rhinitis; include several ways to control environmental allergens.

3. Write a patient teaching plan for the patient with myasthenia gravis.

4. Demonstrate the taking of a detailed history when it is part of the diagnostic work-up in a patient with hypersensitivity illness.

EXERCISES IN FUNDAMENTAL CONCEPTS

1. The word *immune* is derived from the Latin word that means
   "_____."

2. The ability of the immune system to mobilize and use its antibodies and other responses to stimulation by antigen is called
   _____.

3. Immunity is _____
   _____.

4. _____ develop naturally after infection or artificially after vaccinations.

5. Lymphocytes include the T and B cells and the large, granular lymphocytes also known as
   _____.

6. _____ are responsible for cell-mediated immunity and provide the body with protection against viruses, fungi, and parasites.

7. An _____ is a substance recognized as foreign that can trigger an immune response.

8. _____ cause the production of antibodies and proliferate (increase in number) in response to a particular antigen.

9. The process by which resistance to an infectious disease is induced or increased is known as
   _____.

10. When T cells are activated by an antigen, the process known as
    _____ occurs.

11. The complement system is activated when an _____ and an _____ interact.

EXERCISES IN CRITICAL THINKING

Topics for Writing

1. List the 4 R's of the immune response, and describe how each one works.

2. Write a nursing care plan and prioritize the nursing interventions when a patient experiences anaphylaxis.

3. List the major organs of the immune system, and describe how each is involved in the immune response.

4. List the four responses of the immune system, and describe each response.

Topics for Discussion

1. Discuss the difference between natural immunity and acquired immunity.

2. Discuss the roles of T cells and B cells in the immune system, in particular the antigen-antibody reaction.

3. Discuss the mechanisms of the immune response, including cellular immunity.

STUDY QUESTIONS

1. In doing an assessment the nurse knows that the body's first line of defense is:
   a. Specific immunity
   b. Adaptive immunity
   c. Acquired immunity
   d. Nonspecific immunity

2. In assessing immune response the nurse is aware that the T cells, B cells, and NK cells are all:
   a. Platelets
   b. Neutrophils
   c. Lymphocytes
   d. Red blood cells

3. The type of disorder the patient is having when he or she experiences a dramatic reaction to penicillin is:
   a. Urticaria
   b. Dermatitis
   c. Anaphylaxis
   d. Allergic rhinitis

4. The medication most likely to be prescribed for anaphylaxis is:
   a. Demerol
   b. Morphine
   c. Prednisone
   d. Epinephrine

5. When assessing a patient at the onset of severe anaphylaxis reaction, the breath sound that indicates occlusion of the airway is:
   a. Stridor
   b. Crackles
   c. Wheezing
   d. Friction rub

6. If a patient starts wheezing and complaining of chills within 30 minutes after a blood transfusion is started, the nurse:
   a. Calls a code
   b. Gives epinephrine
   c. Stops the transfusion
   d. Notifies the physician

7. Humoral immunity, which is a form of immunity that responds to antigens, is mediated by:
   a. T cells
   b. B cells
   c. NK cells
   d. Phagocytes

8. The patient experiencing an allergic reaction is prescribed an antihistamine to alleviate signs and symptoms. The nurse alerts the patient that this will cause:
   a. Insomnia
   b. Dry cough
   c. Drowsiness
   d. Loss of appetite

9. Each time a person is exposed to an allergen, the allergic response is different. After repeated exposure to an allergen, the chance of a more dramatic allergic reaction is:
   a. None
   b. Lesser
   c. Greater
   d. Possible

10. Terfenadine (Seldane) is often prescribed for allergies because it is less sedating than other antihistamines. It should not be mixed with erythromycin or selected other medications, because it may cause:
    a. Drowsiness
    b. Dysrhythmias
    c. Nasal burning
    d. Urinary retention

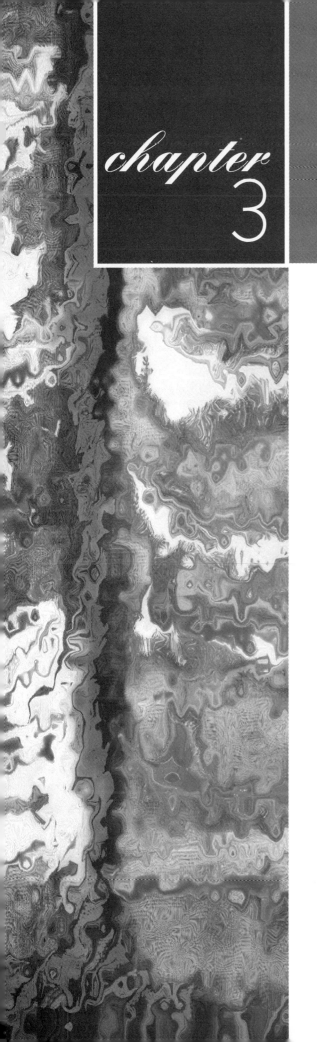

chapter 3

The Surgical Patient

CHAPTER SUMMARY

Chapter 3 presents the nurse's role in the care of the surgical patient beginning with a review of the important assessments and nursing actions during the three phases of the operative process (preoperative, intraoperative, postoperative). Assessment related to IV therapy and blood administration is addressed. Wound healing, signs of infection, and types of wound drainage are described.

LEARNING OBJECTIVES

After reading the chapter in the textbook and working through the chapter in this study guide, the student should be able to do the following:

- Define the key terms found in the matching exercises.
- Identify the purposes for surgery.
- Differentiate among elective, urgent, and emergency surgery.
- Discuss the factors that influence an individual's ability to tolerate surgery.
- Explain the procedure for turnings, deep breathing, coughing, and leg exercises for the postoperative patient.
- Explain the importance of informed consent for surgery.
- Discuss the gerontological considerations for the older adult surgical patient.
- Describe the role of the circulating nurse and the scrub nurse during surgery.
- Discuss the preoperative checklist.
- Discuss the initial nursing assessment and management immediately after transfer from the postanesthesia care unit.

- Identify the rationale for nursing interventions designed to prevent postoperative complications.
- Discuss the nursing process as it pertains to the surgical patient.
- Identify the information needed by the postoperative patient in preparation for discharge.

KEY TERMS AND DEFINITIONS

_____ 1. Ablative
_____ 2. Atelectasis
_____ 3. Catabolism
_____ 4. Dehiscence
_____ 5. Evisceration
_____ 6. Extubate
_____ 7. Exudate
_____ 8. Incentive spirometry
_____ 9. Infarct
_____ 10. Paralytic ileus
_____ 11. Perioperative
_____ 12. Postoperative
_____ 13. Singultus
_____ 14. Surgical asepsis
_____ 15. Thrombus

a. An abnormal condition characterized by the collapse of lung tissue
b. A procedure in which a device is used at the bedside at regular intervals to encourage the patient to deep breathe
c. An involuntary contraction of the diaphragm followed by rapid closure of the glottis
d. The separation of a surgical incision or rupture of a wound closure
e. Entire surgical inpatient period from admission to date of discharge
f. Protection against infection before, during, or after surgery by the use of sterile technique
g. Localized area of necrosis
h. An amputation or excision of any part of the body or removal of a growth or harmful substance
i. Protrusion of an internal organ through a wound or surgical incision, especially in the abdominal wall
j. Period of time after surgery
k. An accumulation of platelets, fibrin, clotting factors, and cellular elements of the blood attached to the anterior wall of a vessel, sometimes occluding the lumen of the vessel
l. A decrease in or absence of intestinal peristalsis that may occur after abdominal surgery, peritoneal trauma, severe metabolic disease, and other conditions
m. Tissue breakdown
n. Fluid, cells, or other substances that have been slowly exuded
o. Removal of an endotracheal tube from an airway

REINFORCING KEY POINTS

1. Discuss the information needed when filling out a preoperative assessment form.

2. Outline the nursing interventions involved in the ABCs of the recovery phase.

3. List the immediate assessments required during the postoperative stage.

4. Explain the difference between the dehiscence and evisceration of a wound.

5. Describe the comfort measures the nurse can implement to decrease pain in the postoperative patient.

6. List the nutritional factors after surgery.

7. Discuss the psychosocial needs of the surgical patient, before and after surgery.

8. Discuss the importance of informed consent.

9. Discuss the factors that affect wound healing.

10. Discuss the nurse's responsibility in assessing wound complications.

11. Differentiate among the following classifications of surgical procedures:
   a. Major

   b. Minor

   c. Elective

   d. Urgent

   e. Palliative

   f. Constructive

12. List the cardinal signs of inflammation/infection.

13. Describe patient teaching for controlled coughing.

14. Discuss the assessments that must be made on the discharge of a surgical patient.

15. Identify what surgery is being performed according to the shaded area below, which represents the area being shaved for surgery preparation:

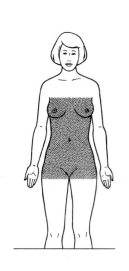

_____

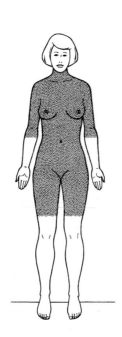

_____

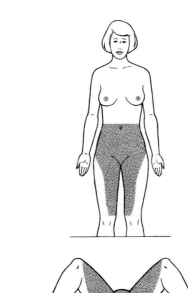

_____

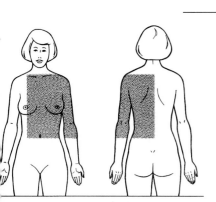

_____

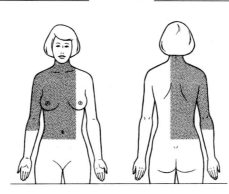

_____

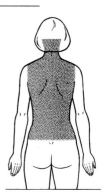

_____

APPLICATION OF CLINICAL SKILLS

1. Describe how to measure for full-length and knee-length antiembolism stockings.

2. Fill out a preoperative assessment form on an imaginary patient.

3. Demonstrate a coughing exercise in preparation to teach a preoperative patient.

4. Teach breathing techniques that are necessary after surgery.

5. Experiment with measuring and applying full-length antiembolism stockings.

EXERCISES IN FUNDAMENTAL CONCEPTS

1. _____ is defined as the branch of medicine concerned with disease and trauma requiring an operative procedure.

2. _____ is an amputation or excision of any part of the body or removal of a growth or harmful substance.

3. _____ therapy is designed to relieve or reduce the intensity of uncomfortable symptoms without cure.

4. _____ refers to the role of the nurse during the preoperative, intraoperative, and postoperative phases of a patient's surgical experience.

5. _____ increases susceptibility to _____ and may _____ from altered glucose metabolism and associated impairment.

6. The patient's bill of rights affirms that the patient must give _____ (permission obtained from a patient to perform a specific test or procedure) before the beginning of any procedure.

EXERCISES IN CRITICAL THINKING

Topics for Writing

1. List the six factors that most influence a patient's surgical experience.

2. List the major considerations to be addressed when preparing a patient for surgery.

3. List the surgeries in which coughing is contraindicated or modified during the postoperative period.

4. Review the ABCs of the recovery period and the nursing interventions involved in each assessment.

5. Describe the seven principles of sterile technique and why each is essential in maintaining surgical asepsis.

Topics for Discussion

1. Discuss the fears most commonly associated with surgery and anesthesia.

2. Discuss how surgery in general affects the major body systems.

3. Discuss the purposes of preoperative teaching and why it is so important.

4. Discuss nursing interventions that will promote comfort and reduce pain for the postoperative patient.

5. Discuss the importance of early ambulation in the postoperative patient.

6. Discuss the physiological factors that affect wound healing and the interventions that can prevent impairment during wound healing.

STUDY QUESTIONS

1. Which of these surgical procedures involves removal of a body organ?
    a. Colostomy
    b. Mammoplasty
    c. Herniorrhaphy
    d. Cholecystectomy

2. Which patient is at great risk for surgical and anesthetic complications?
    a. A 42-year-old scheduled for a breast biopsy
    b. A 3-year-old boy scheduled for a hernia repair
    c. An 80-year-old scheduled for an exploratory laparotomy
    d. An 18-year-old scheduled for an emergency appendectomy

3. Mr. Jensen, an alert 75-year-old man, is to undergo elective surgery. The operative permit must be signed in the presence of a witness by:
    a. Mr. Jensen
    b. Mr. and Mrs. Jensen
    c. Either Mr. or Mrs. Jensen
    d. Mr. Jensen and the surgeon

4. A nursing intervention to assist the patient in coping with fear of pain would be to:
    a. Describe the degree of pain expected
    b. Explain the availability of pain medication
    c. Divert the patient when talking about pain
    d. Inform the patient of the frequency of pain medication

5. The nurse is writing a treatment plan that includes preoperative teaching. The best time to do preoperative teaching is:
    a. 1 week before surgery
    b. 1 to 2 days before surgery
    c. Within 12 hours of surgery
    d. When the preoperative permit is signed

6. The nurse is asked to get an informed consent signed by a patient scheduled for surgery the next morning. The responsibility of the nurse in obtaining informed consent is to:
    a. Explain other options
    b. Explain risks of surgery
    c. Obtain the patient's signature
    d. Check the form for the patient's signature

7. Mr. Jenkins is scheduled for surgery at 6:00 AM. He is asking the nurse, "What is this surgery all about anyway?" The nurse is aware that the legal responsibility for giving information regarding surgery is the responsibility of the:
    a. Aide
    b. Nurse
    c. Hospital
    d. Physician

8. A surgical patient is ordered NPO before surgery. The patient asks, "Why can't I have a drink of water?" The nurse explains that this is a preventive measure for:
    a. Overhydration
    b. Nausea and vomiting
    c. Aspiration pneumonia
    d. Constipation and impaction

9. A patient scheduled for surgery in the morning has the order: "Enemas until clear." Enemas are usually ordered before surgery. The purpose for this is:
    a. To prevent impaction after surgery
    b. To prevent paralytic ileus after surgery
    c. To prevent contamination during surgery
    d. To prevent injury to the colon during surgery

10. Coughing and deep breathing are important in preventing:
    a. Bleeding
    b. Pneumonia
    c. Hypotension
    d. Prolonged pain

11. The action recommended to prevent thrombophlebitis in the postoperative patient at risk for blood clots is:
    a. Leg exercises
    b. Deep breathing
    c. Deep coughing
    d. Splinting for pain

12. Preoperative medication, such as morphine and meperidine (Demerol), is ordered before surgery to:
    a. Eliminate spasms
    b. Enhance the anesthetic
    c. Decrease hypertension
    d. Reduce postoperative pain

13. An 18-month-old child is scheduled to undergo repair and reconstruction of a cleft palate. This surgery is classified as:
    a. Elective
    b. Palliative
    c. Constructive
    d. Reconstructive

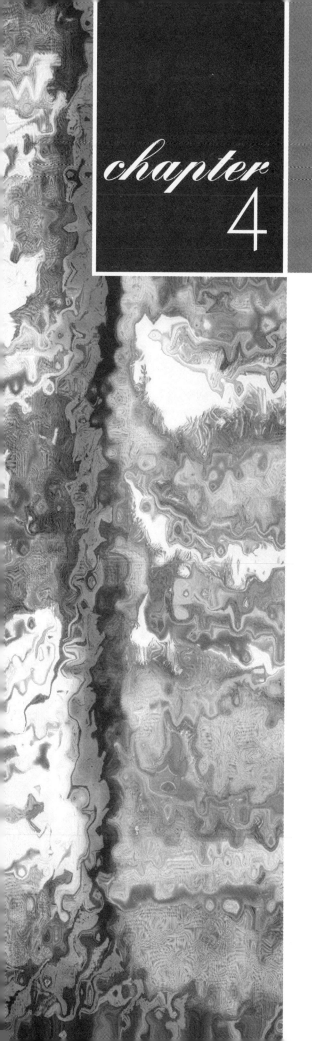

chapter 4

Care of the Patient with an Integumentary Disorder

CHAPTER SUMMARY

Chapter 4 describes the layers of the skin and their functions, with emphasis on nursing interventions for skin disorders. Details on performing a complete skin assessment are outlined. Among the disorders addressed are herpes zoster, impetigo, and tumors of the skin. Care plans are included for patient with shingles, acne, and herpes simplex. Emphasis on care of the burn patient includes medication therapy, skin grafts, and fluid resuscitation. Assessment, including classifications of major burns as well as emergency treatment, and the complications of burns are covered.

LEARNING OBJECTIVES

After reading the chapter in the textbook and studying the chapter in this study guide, the student should be able to do the following:

- Discuss the primary functions of the integumentary system.
- Describe the difference between the epidermis and dermis.
- Discuss the functions of the three major glands located in the skin.
- Define the key terms found in the matching exercises.
- Discuss the general assessment of the skin.
- Identify general nursing interventions for the patient with a skin disorder.

- Discuss how to use the nursing process in caring for patients with skin disorders.
- Discuss viral disorders of the skin.
- Discuss bacterial, fungal, and inflammatory disorders of the skin.
- Identify parasitic disorders of the skin.
- Describe common tumors of the skin.
- Identify disorders associated with the appendages of the skin.
- State the pathologic condition involved in a burn injury.
- Discuss the stages of burn care with appropriate nursing interventions.
- Identify the methods used to classify the extent of a burn injury.

KEY TERMS AND DEFINITIONS

_____	1. Alopecia
_____	2. Contracture
_____	3. Curling's ulcer
_____	4. Heterograft (xenograft)
_____	5. Homograft (allograft)
_____	6. Papule
_____	7. Pustulant vesicles
_____	8. Rule of nines
_____	9. Urticaria
_____	10. Wheal

a. Small, raised, solid skin lesions less than 1 cm in diameter
b. Shortening or tension of muscles that affects extension
c. Divides the body into multiples of nine to measure body area burned
d. Tissue from another species used as a temporary graft
e. Round elevation of the skin, white in the center with a pale red periphery
f. The loss of hair
g. Small, circumscribed elevations of the skin, containing fluid
h. The transfer of tissue between two genetically dissimilar individuals of the same species, such as a skin transplant between two humans who are not identical twins
i. The presence of wheals or hives in an allergic reaction commonly caused by drugs, foods, insect bites, inhalants, emotional stress, or exposure to heat or cold
j. A duodenal ulcer that develops 8 to 14 days after severe burns; the first sign is usually vomiting of bright red blood

REINFORCING KEY POINTS

1. List the major functions of the skin.

2. Name the two layers of skin, and describe how they are different.

3. Describe the following skin lesions:
    a. Ulcer

    b. Wheal

    c. Tumor

    d. Papule

    e. Vesicle

    f. Nodule

    g. Macule

    h. Pustule

4. Discuss the etiology of herpes zoster, or shingles.

5. Describe the lesions found in impetigo.

6. Outline the nursing interventions recommended in treating impetigo.

7. Discuss the assessment and treatment of fungal infections, such as tinea capitis, tinea corporis, tinea cruris, and tinea pedis.

8. State the reasons why contact dermatitis is so common.

9. Discuss the medical management and nursing interventions for urticaria and atopic dermatitis.

10. Differentiate between basal cell carcinoma and squamous cell carcinoma.

11. Describe the factors that determine the depth of a burn injury.

12. Identify how the body is divided into percentages according to the rule of nines in the diagram below:

APPLICATION OF CLINICAL SKILLS

1. Write a teaching plan instructing a mother on how to treat impetigo in an 18-month-old infant.

2. Write a teaching plan for the patient with dermatitis, focusing on relief of itching and discomfort.

3. Instruct a patient regarding the guidelines for baths and therapeutic soaks.

4. Draw a picture of the human body, and designate percentages according to the rule of nines. Do the same for a drawing of a child's body.

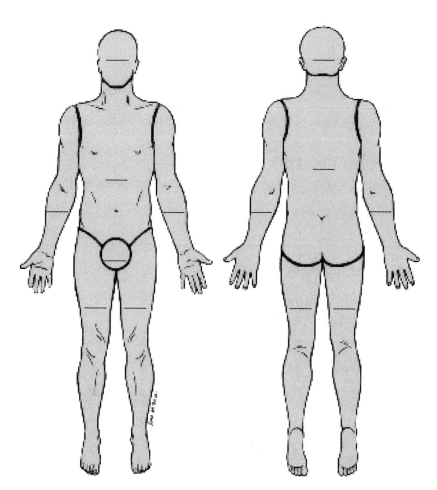

EXERCISES IN FUNDAMENTAL CONCEPTS

1. The _____ is really the body's protector—its first line of defense against infection and injury. In addition to protection, its main function is _____.

2. The skin functions in the prevention and loss of _____ and in the regulation of _____.

3. The inner layer of the epidermis receives its blood supply and nutrition from the underlying dermis through the process of _____.

4. _____ is a black or dark brown pigment that occurs naturally in the hair, skin, and iris and choroid of the eye and is responsible for skin color. Skin color is _____.

5. When the patient has a skin disorder a way to remember to assess the chief complaint is PQRST, which stands for _____, _____, _____, _____, and _____.

6. _____ is decreased oxygen and is indicated by clubbing of the fingertips.

7. Herpes zoster is caused by the chickenpox virus and is commonly known as _____.

EXERCISES IN CRITICAL THINKING

Topics for Writing

1. List gerontological considerations for the older person who is experiencing skin disorders.

2. In a care plan, include patient teaching on the prevention of skin disorders and how to maintain healthy skin.

3. Outline the classification of minor, moderate, and major burns.

Topics for Discussion

1. Discuss the emotional and social impact of a chronic skin disorder and nursing interventions to help the patient cope.

2. Discuss initial emergency treatment in a burn.

3. Discuss the emotional needs of the patient with severe burns.

STUDY QUESTIONS

1. Mrs. Daniels, a nurse, is caring for 18-month-old Danny Allen, who has been diagnosed with impetigo. Patient teaching with the family must emphasize:
   a. It goes away in 3 days
   b. Only children get impetigo
   c. Everyone must take medication
   d. Impetigo is extremely contagious

2. In assessing a Hispanic patient, Mr. Martinez, the nurse notes a yellowish color in the mucous membrane and lips. This is characteristic of:
   a. Pallor
   b. Dry skin
   c. Inflammation
   d. Aging process

3. Mrs. Jones has been diagnosed with herpes zoster (shingles). In planning care, the nurse should take into consideration that Mrs. Jones:
   a. May be very embarrassed
   b. Will be concerned about scarring
   c. Will need large doses of prednisone
   d. Will ask frequently for pain medication

4. The nurse is assessing Mr. Smith, an African-American patient. Mr. Smith has complained of itching and a rash. The rash is not obvious in the area to which Mr. Smith points. To adequately assess his skin, the nurse must:
   a. Order x-rays
   b. Palpate the area
   c. Ask patient to describe the rash
   d. Ask an African-American nurse to do the assessment

5. A patient has been diagnosed with herpes simplex, type I. The drug most likely to be prescribed for this patient is:
   a. Lorazepam (Ativan)
   b. Hydroxyzine (Atarax)
   c. Acyclovir
   d. Erythromycin

6. Mrs. Adams is having intense pain and presents with a painful skin disorder. After assessment the disorder is described as an inflammation along a nerve pathway that produces small skin vesicles. This condition is:
   a. Cellulitis
   b. Pediculosis
   c. Herpes zoster
   d. Herpes simplex

7. An infection surrounding hair follicles is a:
   a. Cellulitis
   b. Carbuncle
   c. Dermatitis
   d. Herpes simplex

8. Amy Evans, 18 months old, has been diagnosed with impetigo. She exhibits the cardinal sign of:
   a. Infected ulcerations on the trunk
   b. Red butterfly rash across the nose
   c. Pustular vesicles with honey-colored crusts
   d. Linear splits and bleeding cracks all over the body

9. The most common fungal infection of the skin is:
   a. Scabies
   b. Tinea pedis
   c. Tinea capitis
   d. Ringworm of the scalp

10. A child has been diagnosed with tinea corporis. The drug prescribed for tinea corporis is:
    a. Lindane (Kwell)
    b. Penicillin
    c. Nystatin (Mycostatin)
    d. Oral griseofulvin

11. A teenage girl is taking isotretinoin (Accutane) for acne. The important precaution during patient teaching that should be emphasized is:
    a. Avoid pregnancy
    b. Avoid acidic foods
    c. Avoid direct sunlight
    d. Avoid other medications

12. A young man presents with a skin disorder characterized by wavy, brownish, threadlike lines. It is determined to be a parasitic condition. This is diagnosed as:
    a. Scabies
    b. Pediculosis
    c. Tinea pedis
    d. Herpes zoster

13. Usually lice are found on children. The medication of choice for pediculosis is:
    a. Lindane (Kwell)
    b. Sulfur
    c. Ampicillin
    d. Petrolatum jelly

14. The following skin tumor is highly malignant:
    a. Melanoma
    b. Actinic keratoses
    c. Basal cell carcinoma
    d. Squamous cell carcinoma

15. Mr. Dallas, an LPN, assesses a white, charred burn on Mr. Bailey, who was involved in a house fire. Mr. Bailey states there is no pain in the area of the burn. Mr. Dallas evaluates this burn as:
    a. Superficial
    b. Full-thickness
    c. Partial-thickness
    d. Deep partial-thickness

16. After a major burn, the patient receiving IV therapy is monitored closely for this possible complication:
    a. Dehydration
    b. Hyperkalemia
    c. Fluid overload
    d. Metabolic alkalosis

17. The most common cause of death in a burn victim during the first 72 hours is:
    a. Infection
    b. Suffocation
    c. Heart attack
    d. Fluid overload

18. Burns that appear dry, red, and blanched on pressure are:
    a. Superficial
    b. Full-thickness
    c. Second-degree
    d. Partial-thickness

19. In assessing burns over the body, the nurse uses the rule of nines as a:
    a. Number of layers necessary to cover burn wound
    b. Formula for determining fluid volume replacement
    c. Formula for determining amount of skin area burned
    d. Comparison of body surface burned with patient's age

20. Pigskin is the following type of skin graft:
    a. Autograft
    b. Homograft
    c. Heterograft
    d. Synthetic graft

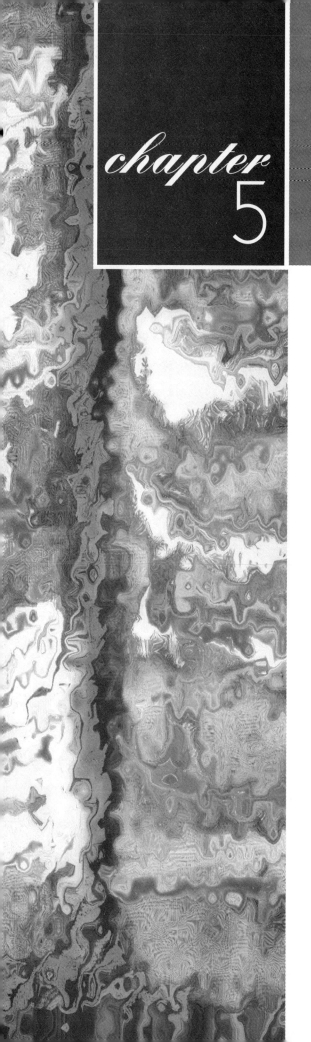

chapter 5

Care of the Patient with a Musculoskeletal Disorder

CHAPTER SUMMARY

Chapter 5 reviews the basic functions of the skeletal system. The bones and muscles are listed and described. Detailed assessments of the musculoskeletal and neuromuscular systems along with appropriate nursing interventions are described. Musculoskeletal disorders (e.g., arthritis, osteoporosis, ankylosing spondylitis) are presented. Serious complications (e.g., fat embolism, shock, compartment syndrome, thromboembolus) are outlined in detail.

LEARNING OBJECTIVES

After reading the chapter in the textbook and working through the chapter in this study guide, the student should be able to do the following:

Anatomy and Physiology
- Define the key terms found in the matching exercises.
- List five basic functions of the skeletal system.
- List two divisions of the skeleton.
- Describe the location of major bones of the skeleton.
- Describe three vital functions that muscles perform when they contract.
- List the types of body movements.

Medical-Surgical

- Describe the following conditions: lordosis, scoliosis, and kyphosis.
- Describe five diagnostic procedures pertinent to musculoskeletal function.
- Compare methods for assessing circulation, nerve damage, and infection in a patient who has received a traumatic insult to the musculoskeletal system.
- List at least four healthy lifestyle measures a person can practice to reduce the risk of developing osteoporosis.
- List at least two types of skin and skeletal traction.
- List four nursing interventions appropriate for patients with bone cancer.
- Describe the phenomenon of phantom pain.
- Compare the medical regimen for patients with "gouty" arthritis, rheumatoid arthritis, and osteoarthritis.
- Discuss the nursing interventions appropriate for patients with rheumatoid arthritis.
- Describe the nursing interventions appropriate for degenerative joint disease (osteoarthritis and ankylosing spondylitis).
- Describe the surgical intervention for arthritis of the hip and knee.
- Describe the symptoms of compartment syndrome.
- Discuss the physiology of fracture healing (hematoma, granulation tissue, and callus formation).
- Discuss nursing interventions appropriate for a patient with a fractured hip after ORIF or bipolar hip prosthesis.
- Describe the nursing interventions for the patient undergoing a total hip or a total knee replacement.

KEY TERMS AND DEFINITIONS

_____ 1. Acetabulum
_____ 2. Arthrocentesis
_____ 3. Articulation
_____ 4. Compartment syndrome
_____ 5. Crepitus
_____ 6. Foramen magnum
_____ 7. Gait
_____ 8. Ischium
_____ 9. Ligament
_____ 10. Lordosis
_____ 11. Paresthesia
_____ 12. Scoliosis
_____ 13. Tendon
_____ 14. Traction

a. One of many predominantly white, shiny, flexible bands of fibrous tissue binding joints together and connecting various bones and cartilages
b. Manner or style of walking
c. A pathogenic condition caused by the progressive development of arterial vessel compression and reduced blood supply to an extremity
d. Puncture of a joint with a needle to withdraw fluid
e. Abnormal lateral or S curvature of the spine
f. Numbness, weakness, or a tingling sensation
g. Passage in the occipital bone through which the spinal cord enters the spinal column
h. One of the three parts of the hip bone, joining the ilium and the pubis to form the acetabulum
i. Having a limb, bone, or group of muscles under tension with weights and pulleys; aligns or immobilizes the part and relieves pressure on it
j. One of many white, glistening, fibrous bands of tissue that attach muscle to bone
k. Increased curve in the lumbar region of the spine
l. A grating sound heard on movement of ends of a broken bone
m. The large, cup-shaped articular cavity at the junction of the ilium, the ischium, and the pubis, containing the ball-shaped head of the femur
n. Gliding, rotation, and angular movement of a joint

REINFORCING KEY POINTS

1. Describe the five basic functions of the skeletal system.

2. Describe the three vital functions that muscles perform.

3. Explain the "all or none" law of muscles.

4. Discuss how a neurotransmitter stimulates muscle fiber.

5. Describe the nine types of body movement.

6. Describe the purpose of a doppler.

7. Describe the blanching test.

8. Differentiate among kyphosis, lordosis, and scoliosis.

9. Name the three purposes for which arthroscopy might be ordered.

10. Discuss the pathophysiology and clinical manifestations of osteoarthritis.

11. Discuss the etiology and medical management of osteoporosis.

12. Differentiate between a strain and a sprain.

13. Differentiate between the following fractures by giving an example:
    a. Spiral

    b. Oblique

    c. Impacted

    d. Complete

e. Greenstick

f. Transverse

g. Comminuted

14. Discuss the five complications of fractures and important nursing assessments of each.

15. Discuss the various aspects of patient care for a patient in a cast.

16. Give the six purposes for which traction is ordered.

17. Differentiate between skeletal and skin traction, and give examples of each.

18. Review the nursing interventions necessary when a patient is in traction.

19. Outline the nursing interventions required for the patient undergoing total knee replacement.

20. Discuss postoperative interventions required for the person with an amputation.

21. Identify the fractures in the figure below:

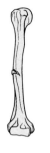 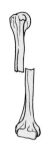 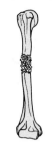

_____ _____ _____

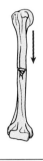 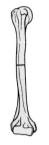

_____ _____

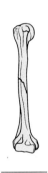 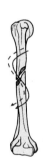

_____ _____

APPLICATION OF CLINICAL SKILLS

1. Write a teaching plan for the patient who has had a hip prosthetic implant.

2. Cite the priority nursing interventions in these complications of fractures:
   a. Shock
   b. Fat embolism
   c. Gas gangrene
   d. Thromboembolus
   e. Compartment syndrome

3. Demonstrate how the "all or none" law governs muscles.

4. Demonstrate neurovascular checks.

5. Teach a mother how to assess for scoliosis in her young daughter.

6. Teach a patient with arthritis about the precautions that should be taken when aspirin is prescribed.

7. Show a patient with an ankle sprain how to wrap an Ace bandage with the figure-of-8 wrap.

8. Explain to the patient in a cast the care required and the rationale for each intervention; emphasize how the patient can help to maintain optimal skin integrity.

9. Demonstrate how to walk on crutches, describing the two-point gait, the three-point gait, and the four-point gait.

EXERCISES IN FUNDAMENTAL CONCEPTS

1. The skeletal system has five basic functions:
   _____, _____, _____,
   _____, and _____.

2. _____ is blood cell formation and takes place in the red bone marrow.

3. There are four classifications of the bones, based on their form and shape: _____, _____, _____, and _____.

4. Muscle tissue is under voluntary or involuntary control. Voluntary muscle is _____, whereas involuntary muscle tissue responds to _____.

5. Muscle cells, in union with the nerve cells that control them, are called a _____.

6. The impulse from the nerve cell must travel across a small gap, since the nerve cell and the muscle cell do not directly touch each other. This small gap is called a _____ .

7. A special chemical that travels through the fluid to stimulate the muscle fiber is called a _____.

8. _____ is the specific neurotransmitter for the skeletal muscle tissue.

9. Muscle cells are governed by the "_____" law, which states that when a muscle cell is adequately stimulated or shocked, it will contract completely.

10. Skeletal muscles are usually classified into two broad categories: _____ and _____.

11. The _____ muscle groups are those muscles located on the head, face, neck, and trunk.

12. The _____ muscle groups are all the muscles of the extremities.

13. The musculoskeletal system provides _____, _____, and _____.

14. Circulatory status is assessed by signs of _____, _____, _____, and _____.

15. A test of the rate of capillary refill, which signals circulation status, is called _____.

16. A circulation check is also known as a _____ and includes assessment of _____, _____, and _____.

17. Remember the 5 P's when conducting a neurovascular assessment:
    a. _____
    b. _____
    c. _____
    d. _____
    e. _____

EXERCISES IN CRITICAL THINKING

Topics for Writing

1. Photocopy an unlabeled picture of a skeleton with muscles, and note the major bones of the body.

2. Do the same as above, and note the major muscle groups of the body.

3. Discuss the implications of the 5 P's in a neuromuscular assessment.

4. Outline the essentials of a neurovascular assessment and the rationale for each.

Topics for Discussion

1. Discuss the difference between rheumatoid arthritis and osteoarthritis.

2. Discuss the difference between a sprain and a strain and the nursing implications for each.

3. Discuss the immediate nursing management required when a bone is fractured.

4. Discuss the gerontological considerations when caring for an elderly person with an orthopedic injury.

5. Discuss the potential complications that a nurse must assess when caring for a patient with a fracture, especially a neurovascular assessment.

STUDY QUESTIONS

1. Hemopoiesis, or the formation of blood cells, takes place in the:
   a. Liver
   b. Spleen
   c. Flat, long bones
   d. Red bone marrow

2. The hip socket, formed by the hip bones, is called the:
   a. Ischium
   b. Acromion
   c. Olecranon
   d. Acetabulum

3. The projection of cartilage at the lower border of the sternum is called the:
   a. Xiphoid process
   b. Acromion process
   c. Olecranon process
   d. Zygomatic process

4. The bands of connective tissue that bind the joints together and anchor muscles to bones are called:
   a. Bursa
   b. Fascia
   c. Ligaments
   d. Tendon sheaths

5. The bone that forms the back of the skull is the:
   a. Ethmoid
   b. Occipital
   c. Sphenoid
   d. Temporal

6. In performing a neurovascular check on Mrs. Stevens, 24 years old, who has been treated for a fractured arm, the nurse notes the tissue color is blanched and white. This indicates:
   a. Venous stasis
   b. Increased blood supply
   c. Poorly oxygenated tissue
   d. Fluid accumulating in tissues

7. Mrs. Jones, 32 years old, has just been diagnosed with rheumatoid arthritis. Acute rheumatoid arthritis is characterized by a pathological process in the joint called:
   a. Fusion
   b. Degeneration
   c. Inflammation
   d. Bone spur growth

8. Mrs. Jones's chief complaint (and the most common problem of rheumatoid arthritis) is:
   a. Fever and pain
   b. Inability to move
   c. Stiffness in the morning
   d. Limited joint movement

9. Mr. Davis, 34 years old, is suffering back strain and inflammation. He is prescribed a non-steroidal antiinflammatory agent. He is taking:
   a. Aspirin
   b. Acetaminophen (Tylenol)
   c. Prednisone
   d. Phenylbutazone (Butazolidin)

10. Mrs. Jones is prescribed a medication for rheumatoid arthritis. One of the most common side effects of medications prescribed for rheumatoid arthritis is:
    a. Skin rash
    b. Dizziness
    c. Fluid retention
    d. Gastric irritation

11. Mr. Daniel sprained his ankle 4 hours before coming to the emergency room. The physician has ordered the diagnostic study most common for determining musculoskeletal integrity. Mr. Daniel is scheduled for a (an):
    a. Magnetic resonance imaging (MRI)
    b. X-ray
    c. Computed tomography (CT) scan
    d. Bone scan

12. Mrs. Peterson, 21 years old, has been involved in a car accident, and x-rays have been ordered for her arms and legs. An important question to ask Mrs. Peterson before the x-rays are taken is:
    a. "Are you having intense pain?"
    b. "Has your head been injured?"
    c. "Can you move your arms and legs?"
    d. "Is there any possibility that you might be pregnant?"

13. Mr. Simmons, 38 years old, is scheduled for a myelogram following an on-the-job work injury in which he injured his lower back. The nurse tells him he has been scheduled for a myelogram. He states the physician told him a needle will be inserted into his spine and he is afraid that it might paralyze him. The nurse alleviates this fear by telling him:
    a. "I think you worried for nothing."
    b. "No one has ever suffered this complication."
    c. "You have a valid concern, but that would be rare."
    d. "The spinal cord ends above the area where the needle will go."

14. Mrs. Fielder, 34 years old, is scheduled to undergo an MRI to detect a herniated nucleus pulposus. The nurse must caution Mrs. Fielder:
    a. That the test can be extremely painful
    b. To do progressive muscle relaxation exercises
    c. That the test will take 24 hours to fully complete
    d. To take off all jewelry, glasses, and anything made with metal

15. Mrs. Jensen, 68 years old, is scheduled for a CT scan. The nurse asks her if she is allergic to seafood or iodine. Mrs. Jensen replies, "My, you ask some strange questions." The nurse replies:
    a. "I know, but the doctor wants all of this information."
    b. "It's important to have a very thorough medical history."
    c. "This might change the medication we give you during the test."
    d. "This will help to detect allergy to the medication used in this test."

16. Mr. Cousins, 56 years old, has been diagnosed with ankylosing spondylitis. The physician states he has had the disease for some time. Ankylosing spondylitis often goes undiagnosed because:
    a. There are no laboratory tests for diagnosis
    b. It is a painless disease that lasts 20 years
    c. Low back pain and sciatica are the first symptoms
    d. It takes 20 years for signs to become obvious

17. Mrs. Dennis, 68 years old, has been diagnosed with osteoarthritis. Osteoarthritis is most often associated with:
    a. Inflammatory process
    b. Previous bone disease
    c. Genetic predisposition
    d. Degeneration, with age

18. Reconstruction of a joint that has been destroyed by disease is termed:
    a. Osteotomy
    b. Arthrodesis
    c. Arthrotomy
    d. Arthroplasty

19. Mrs. Beebe has Heberden's nodes in her hands. They are commonly seen in this disorder:
    a. Osteoarthritis
    b. Bacterial arthritis
    c. Rheumatoid arthritis
    d. Carpal tunnel syndrome

20. The physician is likely to prescribe the following medication for the patient with osteoarthritis:
    a. Oxycodone and acetaminophen (Tylox)
    b. Aspirin
    c. Codeine
    d. Acetaminophen (Tylenol #3)

21. Mrs. Billings suffered a fracture of the tibia in a car accident. A fracture in which the bone has broken into several fragments is called:
    a. Greenstick
    b. Pathological
    c. Compound
    d. Comminuted

22. Mrs. Ingram, 67 years old, underwent a total hip replacement 6 hours ago. In caring for her, the nurse is aware that the leg position that must be avoided for up to 2 months after total hip replacement is:
    a. Extension
    b. Abduction
    c. Adduction
    d. Knee flexion

23. A precaution to be taken when a patient has a compound fracture is:
    a. Buck's traction at the fracture site
    b. No narcotics for pain
    c. Tetanus immunization
    d. Sterile gauze application

24. A patient who suffered a fracture 2 days ago is now experiencing dyspnea, chest pain, and confusion. The nurse takes precautions against the following complication:
    a. Osteomyelitis
    b. Fat embolism
    c. Ischemic paralysis
    d. Acute bone infection

25. Traction by straight pull on a traction boot applied to an extended leg is termed:
    a. Buck's traction
    b. Russell traction
    c. Skeletal traction
    d. Balanced suspension

26. In preparing a patient for a myelogram, it is imperative for the nurse to inform the patient that the procedure will be in the lumbar region, below the spinal cord, at the level of:
    a. L1
    b. L2
    c. L3
    d. L4, L5

27. An important nursing intervention for the patient during the first hours following a myelo-gram is to:
   a. Sit upright
   b. Force fluids
   c. Ambulate early
   d. Keep medicated

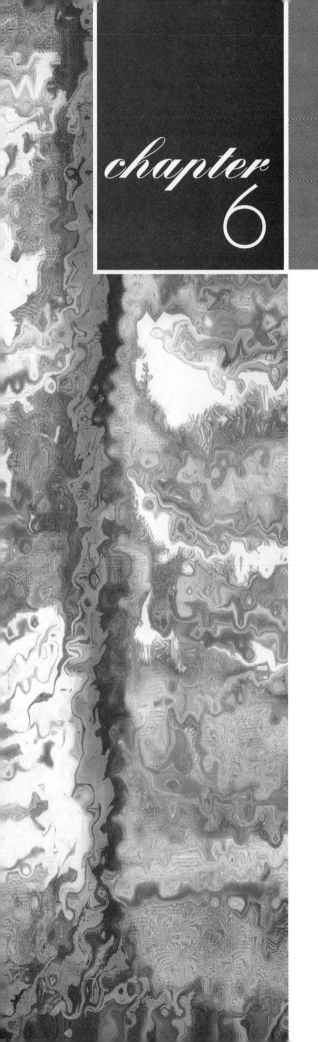

chapter 6

Care of the Patient with a Gastrointestinal Disorder

CHAPTER SUMMARY

Chapter 6 reviews the anatomy and physiology of the digestive system to help the student understand how the gastrointestinal (GI) tract works. Assessments of the GI system and diagnostic tests for the most common disorders are described. Nursing interventions for conditions such as peptic ulcers, ulcerative colitis, irritable bowel syndrome, Crohn's disease, and cancer of the stomach are detailed. The most common nursing interventions are highlighted in easy-to-read charts. The nurse's responsibility in surgical procedures, such as gastric resection, cancer of the colon, and intestinal obstruction, are outlined.

LEARNING OBJECTIVES

After reading the chapter in the textbook and working through the chapter in this study guide, the student should be able to do the following:

Anatomy and Physiology
- List in sequence each of the component parts of the alimentary canal, and identify the accessory organs of digestion.
- Discuss the functions of each digestive and accessory organ.

Medical-Surgical

- Define the key terms found in the matching exercises.
- Discuss nursing interventions for six diagnostic examinations for patients with disorders of the GI tract.
- Explain the common causes, clinical manifestations, diagnosis, medical-surgical management, and nursing interventions for the patient with peptic ulcer disease.
- Describe the clinical manifestations, medical-surgical management, and nursing interventions for the patient with cancer of the stomach.
- Identify nursing interventions for preoperative and postoperative care for the patient with gastric resection.
- Differentiate between diverticulosis and diverticulitis, including medical management and nursing interventions.
- Compare and contrast the types of hernias, including etiology and surgical and nursing interventions.
- Describe the clinical manifestations, surgical procedures, and nursing interventions for the patient with cancer of the colon and rectum.
- Identify five nursing interventions for the patient with a stoma for fecal diversion.

a. An artificial opening of an internal organ on the surface of the body
b. Increase in the severity of the disease or any of its symptoms
c. Weakness and emaciation associated with general ill health and malnutrition
d. A white, firmly attached patch on the mouth or tongue mucosa
e. Blood that is obscure or hidden from view, usually found in feces
f. An abnormal condition characterized by the inability of the muscle to relax, particularly the cardiac sphincter of the stomach
g. Excess fat in the feces
h. Infolding of one segment of the intestine into the lumen of another segment
i. A glycoprotein antigen in adenocarcinomas of the GI tract
j. Tarlike, fetid-smelling stool containing undigested blood
k. A surgical joining of two ducts or blood vessels to allow flow from one to the other
l. A partial or complete separation of wound edges

KEY TERMS AND DEFINITIONS

_____	1. Achalasia
_____	2. Anastomosis
_____	3. Cachexia
_____	4. Carcinoembryonic antigen
_____	5. Dehiscence
_____	6. Exacerbation
_____	7. Intussusception
_____	8. Leukoplakia
_____	9. Melena
_____	10. Occult blood
_____	11. Steatorrhea
_____	12. Stoma

REINFORCING KEY POINTS

1. Identify the location of the digestive organs in the figure below:

2. List the functions of the accessory organs.

3. State the purpose of an endoscopy and the essential body function that the nurse must assess following the procedure of endoscopy.

4. Discuss the purpose of the upper GI series and the nursing interventions required for a successful test.

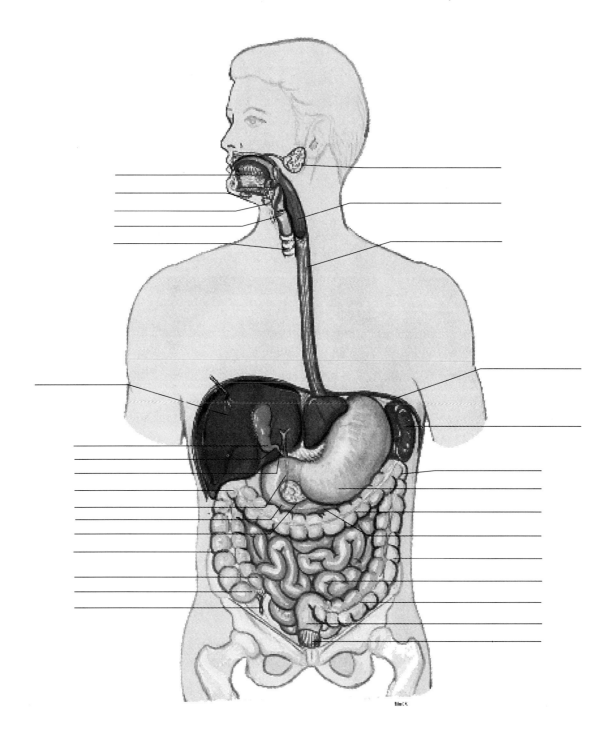

5. Discuss the nursing interventions for the patient scheduled to undergo a barium swallow.

6. Discuss the medical and nursing management that is required for the treatment of candidiasis.

7. Discuss the medical and nursing management for a patient who has cancer of the mouth.

8. List the medications that are often prescribed for the person with gastritis.

9. Discuss the etiology and treatment of peptic and duodenal ulcers.

10. List the drugs of choice for ulcers.

11. Describe the dumping syndrome and how this complication is treated.

12. Describe what is involved in gastric and intestinal suctioning care.

13. Outline the subjective and objective data that the nurse would find in the patient who has cancer of the stomach.

14. Discuss the etiology of these intestinal disorders:
    a. Crohn's disease

    b. Ulcerative colitis

    c. Intestinal infections

15. List the signs and symptoms of appendicitis.

16. Discuss the medical and nursing management for the patient with cancer of the colon.

17. Discuss the etiology and clinical manifestations of hemorrhoids.

18. Discuss dietary considerations for the patient with hemorrhoids.

19. Cite the complications the nurse watches for after a colonoscopy.

APPLICATION OF CLINICAL SKILLS

1. Consider patient teaching plans for the following disorders:
   a. Ulcerative colitis
   b. Irritable bowel syndrome
   c. Crohn's disease

2. Note the priority interventions for a patient suffering an intestinal obstruction.

3. Write a nursing care plan for the patient scheduled for a gastric resection.

4. Write a patient teaching care plan for the patient with a peptic ulcer, emphasizing dietary aspects.

5. Describe maintenance of a nasogastric tube.

6. Cite the purposes of nasogastric intubation.

7. Describe the procedure involved in colostomy, ileostomy, and urostomy care.

8. Describe the procedure for performing colostomy irrigation.

9. Describe the emergency medical treatment required when esophageal varices rupture.

10. Describe the procedure for gastric lavage.

11. Instruct the patient with diverticular disease about what diet is recommended.

12. Write a teaching plan for the patient with hemorrhoids, including nutritional measures that are recommended.

EXERCISES IN FUNDAMENTAL CONCEPTS

1. The _____ is a musculomembranous tube extending from the mouth to the anus and is approximately 30 feet long.

2. The entrance to the stomach is the _____ (so named because of the proximity to the heart); the exit is the _____.

3. The inner surface of the small intestine contains millions of tiny, fingerlike projections clustered over the entire mucous surface called _____.

4. The liver is the largest glandular organ in the body and one of the most complex. It is located just _____ _____.

5. The _____ contains two centers that affect eating. One center stimulates the individual to eat, and the other signals the individual to stop eating.

6. The _____ is an acid-perfusion test that is used to reproduce the symptoms of gastroesophageal reflux. It aids in differentiating esophageal pain caused by esophageal reflux from that caused by _____.

7. _____ is a fungal organism normally present in the mucous membrane of the _____, _____, and _____. Candidiasis appears as small white patches on the mucous membranes of the mouth and the tongue.

8. Kaposi's sarcoma is a malignant skin tumor that is seen as a nonsquamous lesion in patients with _____. These lesions are purple and nonulcerated.

EXERCISES IN CRITICAL THINKING

Topics for Writing

1. Label the quadrants in the abdominal cavity, and list the major organs in each quadrant.

2. In a care plan for an older adult with GI bleeding, outline the gerontological considerations when an older adult is experiencing GI problems.

Topics for Discussion

1. Discuss how the intake of food is regulated in the body and how eating patterns are balanced.

2. Discuss the effects of metabolism on the body and how it can be controlled.

3. Discuss the psychological impact of GI disorders, particularly ulcers and colitis.

STUDY QUESTIONS

1. Mr. Justin is scheduled for a tube gastric analysis. A hold is put on anticholinergic medications. The rationale for this is that anticholinergic medications will:
   a. Change gastric flora
   b. Cause many side effects
   c. Alter gastric acid secretion
   d. Inhibit placement of a nasogastric tube

2. Mrs. Smith is scheduled for a colonoscopy. In preparing Mrs. Smith for this test, the nurse instructs her to drink a solution of GoLYTELY. She cautions her to drink it:
   a. Slowly
   b. Quickly
   c. At 1- to 2-hour intervals
   d. At 30-minute intervals

3. Mr. Gates has been admitted to the hospital with cancer of the esophagus. The nurse performs a careful oral assessment because:
   a. Cancer turns the tongue black
   b. Dysphagia is a common symptom
   c. There is a correlation between cancer and dental caries
   d. There is a high correlation between cancer of the mouth and cancer of the esophagus

4. During an initial assessment the nurse notes a lesion in Mr. Dennis's mouth; the following pre-malignant lesion has the highest potential for malignancy:
   a. Thrush
   b. Leukoplakia
   c. Erythroplasia
   d. Erythroplakia

5. In the morning during patient teaching, Mrs. Davis is scheduled to have a barium enema. The nurse instructs Mrs. Davis that after the barium enema she will be assessed for:
   a. Gastric discomfort
   b. Cardiac abnormalities
   c. Blood in the barium of the enema
   d. Complete evacuation of the barium

6. The nurse assesses white patches, like milk curds, over inflamed tissue in the mouth. This is called:
   a. Gingivitis
   b. Candidiasis
   c. Periodontitis
   d. Herpetic stomatitis

7. The nurse is teaching a GI patient about digestion. She explains that normal passage of the food through the stomach, small intestine, and large intestine takes:
   a. 24 hours
   b. 48 hours
   c. 2 to 3 days
   d. 3 to 5 days

8. When a patient is diagnosed with an ulcer, the nurse teaches that the major complication of a gastric ulcer is:
   a. Strict dietary restrictions
   b. Sudden hemorrhaging of ulcer
   c. Restricted, low-stress lifestyle
   d. Taking medications for a lifetime

9. A patient hospitalized with an ulcer begins to vomit "coffee-ground" vomitus. This is indicative of:
   a. Fresh bleeding
   b. Blood, partly digested
   c. Excessive bile secretion
   d. Contents from an obstruction

10. Mrs. Lawson has been diagnosed with diverticulosis caused by increased intracolonic pressure. The nurse instructs her on a diet of:
    a. High calories, low fiber
    b. High protein, high calories
    c. High carbohydrates, low protein
    d. High fiber (bran, fruits, vegetables)

11. The nurse is assessing a patient with a nasogastric tube. The most accurate method of determining that a nasogastric tube is in the stomach is to take the end of the tube and:
    a. Hold it under water; watch for bubbling
    b. Attach a syringe; aspirate gastric contents
    c. Insert 10 ml of water; listen for airflow with a stethoscope
    d. Insert 2 ml of sterile water; listen for gurgling with stethoscope

12. In teaching a patient with inflammatory bowel disease the emphasis is on nutrition. The diet should be high in:
    a. Milk, eggs
    b. Calories, protein
    c. Vitamins, minerals
    d. Simple carbohydrates

13. In assessing the patient with abdominal pain, it should be noted that the pain of appendicitis is often located midway between the umbilicus and the:
    a. Left ileum
    b. Right ilcum
    c. Left lower rib cage
    d. Right lower rib cage

14. The patient experiencing appendicitis has pain, nausea, and rebound tenderness in the lower right quadrant; the objective data that will be seen are:
    a. Rigid abdomen, fever
    b. Increased red blood cell count (RBC), high fever
    c. Decreased white blood cell count (WBC), hypotension
    d. Increased WBC, low-grade fever

15. The cause of diverticulosis is unknown, but one risk factor is:
    a. Aspirin
    b. Smoking
    c. Low-fiber diet
    d. High-fiber diet

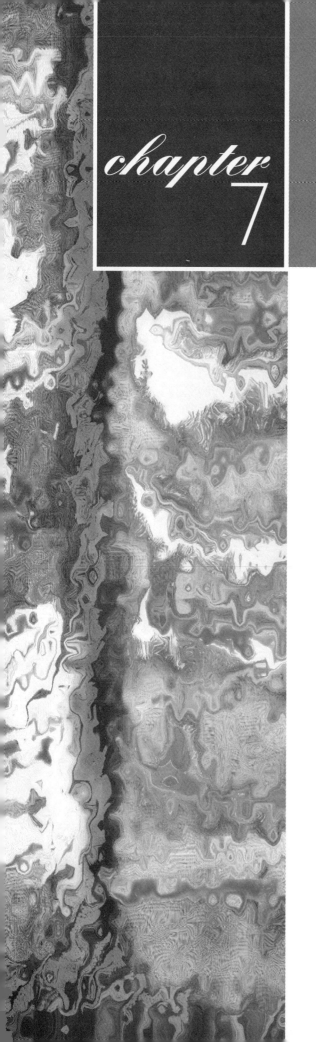

chapter 7

Care of the Patient with an Accessory Organ Disorder

CHAPTER SUMMARY

Chapter 7 discusses the nursing assessment and interventions for patients with disorders of the accessory organs. The chapter details the diagnostic examinations and tests related to these diagnoses, which include viral hepatitis, cirrhosis of the liver, pancreatitis, and cancer of the pancreas. The clinical manifestations and surgical management for the patient with gallbladder disorders are detailed.

LEARNING OBJECTIVES

After reading the chapter in the textbook and working through the chapter in this study guide, the student should be able to do the following:

- Define the key terms found in the matching exercises.
- Discuss nursing interventions for the diagnostic examinations for patients with disorders of the accessory organs.
- Define jaundice, and describe other signs and symptoms that may occur with jaundice.
- State the five types of viral hepatitis, including the modes of transmission.
- List the subjective and objective data for the patient with viral hepatitis.
- Explain the etiology, pathophysiology, clinical manifestations, complications, medical management, and nursing interventions for the patient with cirrhosis of the liver.

- Discuss specific teaching content for the patient with cirrhosis of the liver.
- Explain the clinical manifestations and medical management and nursing interventions for the patient with acute pancreatitis and chronic pancreatitis.
- Explain the clinical manifestations, medical management, and nursing interventions for the patient with carcinoma of the pancreas.
- Explain the etiology, pathophysiology, clinical manifestations, and medical and surgical management for the patient with gallbladder disorders.

KEY TERMS AND DEFINITIONS

_____ 1. Ascites
_____ 2. Asterixis
_____ 3. Esophageal varices
_____ 4. Flatulence
_____ 5. Hepatic encephalopathy
_____ 6. Hepatitis
_____ 7. Jaundice
_____ 8. Occlusion
_____ 9. Paracentesis
_____ 10. Parenchyma
_____ 11. Steatorrhea

a. A hand-flapping tremor that is usually induced by extending the arm and dorsiflexing the wrist; seen frequently in hepatic coma
b. An accumulation of fluid and albumin in the peritoneal cavity
c. A type of brain damage caused by liver disease and consequent ammonia intoxication
d. Excessive fat in the feces
e. An obstruction or closing off
f. A complex of longitudinal, tortuous veins at the lower end of the esophagus
g. Yellow discoloration of the skin, mucous membrane, and sclera of eyes, caused by greater than normal amounts of bilirubin in the blood
h. Tissue of an organ, as distinguished from supporting or connective tissue
i. Excess formation of gases in the stomach or intestine
j. A procedure in which fluid is withdrawn from the abdominal cavity by either gravity or vacuum
k. An inflammation of the liver resulting from bacterial agents or exposure to a toxic substance

REINFORCING KEY POINTS

1. Discuss the rationale for enzyme tests when liver, gallbladder, and pancreatic disorders are diagnosed.

2. Discuss the nursing interventions when a patient is scheduled for a liver biopsy.

3. Discuss the effects of cirrhosis of the liver, including the course of the disease and medical management.

4. Discuss hepatic encephalopathy, including the cause, nursing interventions, and prognosis.

5. Discuss the different types of hepatitis and how they are spread.

6. Identify the duodenum, stab wound, T tube, hepatic ducts, cystic duct stump, common bile duct, and pancreatic duct in the figure below:

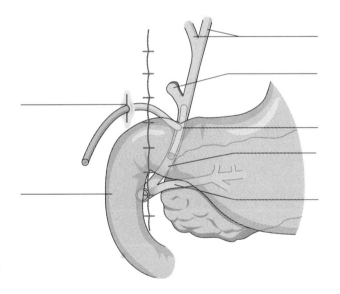

APPLICATION OF CLINICAL SKILLS

1. Describe the nursing interventions, including patient teaching, for the patient who is scheduled for a liver biopsy.

2. Describe nursing interventions for the patient who is scheduled for a computed tomography (CT) scan of the abdomen.

3. Describe the several modes of transmission of the five types of hepatitis and how to prevent each mode of transmission.

EXERCISES IN FUNDAMENTAL CONCEPTS

1. Although elevation of serum enzymes is found in pathological liver conditions, the tests are not

   _____.

2. One way to assess the functional status of the liver is to measure the

   _____.

3. Ascites is the _____.

4. _____ is a procedure in which fluid is withdrawn from the abdominal cavity that will relieve ascites and also provide fluid for laboratory examination.

5. _____ is an inflammation of the liver resulting from several causes, including viral agents, bacterial agents, or exposure to toxic substances.

EXERCISES IN CRITICAL THINKING

Topics for Writing

1. Draw a pathway covering the etiology, pathophysiology, and nursing interventions for a patient diagnosed with cirrhosis.

2. Write a care plan for a patient who is scheduled for a laparoscopic cholecystectomy.

Topics for Discussion

1. Describe how alcohol gradually affects the body, especially the liver.

2. Discuss nursing interventions following a paracentesis, especially considering emotional support of the patient.

STUDY QUESTIONS

1. Mr. Billings is scheduled for a gallbladder series and cholecystogram in the morning. An important nursing intervention before the tablets are administered is:
   a. Instruct patient to void
   b. Give a cleansing enema
   c. Begin an IV line of normal saline
   d. Careful assessment for allergies

2. The physician has ordered a liver biopsy on Mr. Davis, 48 years old, who has stated that he has been an alcoholic for 20 years. Before the procedure is performed the nurse must make sure that the following laboratory test or tests have been done and results reported to the physician:
   a. Blood glucose level
   b. Alcohol blood levels
   c. Platelet and prothrombin
   d. Aspartate transaminase (AST), alanine (ALA), and K-glutamyltransferase (GGT)

3. A blood ammonia test has been ordered for Mr. Simmons, 38 years old, whose symptoms indicate severe liver dysfunction. On the requisition the nurse must be careful to note:
   a. History of hepatitis
   b. His weight and age
   c. If he is an alcoholic
   d. Antibiotics he is taking

4. Mr. Dawson, who has had symptoms of pancreatitis, is scheduled for a urine amylase test. The nurse must be careful to:
   a. Instruct him to avoid drinking caffeine
   b. Cancel the test if symptoms subside
   c. Instruct him to be NPO for 24 hours
   d. Record the beginning and ending of the test

5. Mr. Nelson is scheduled to undergo an endoscopic retrograde cholangiopancreatogram (ERCP) of the pancreatic duct. The nurse is asking him to sign an informed consent for the procedure. She instructs Mr. Nelson that during the test it is very important for him to:
   a. Show no signs of pain
   b. Lie completely motionless
   c. Call for help if pain intensifies
   d. Take plenty of pain medication

6. Mr. Rhodes has been diagnosed with cirrhosis of the liver. He is placed on a low-fat, low-salt diet that is also:
   a. High-fat, high-sodium
   b. High-calorie, high-protein
   c. High in fluids and protein
   d. Low-calorie, low-salt, low-fat

7. Mr. Rhodes is suffering nausea and vomiting. The physician orders an antiemetic. The nurse prepares to administer:
   a. Hydroxyzine (Atarax)
   b. Hydroxyzine (Vistaril)
   c. Diphenhydramine (Benadryl)
   d. Prochlorperazine (Compazine)

8. Mr. Stevens has ascites secondary to cirrhosis. To obtain diuresis the physician orders:
   a. Spironolactone (Aldactone)
   b. Dopamine
   c. Prochlorperazine (Compazine)
   d. Furosemide (Lasix) IV push

9. The cause of cirrhosis of the liver in the Western world is:
   a. Trauma
   b. Alcohol
   c. Drug toxicity
   d. Viral inflammation

10. The following assessment requires ongoing monitoring for the patient with cirrhosis of the liver:
    a. Vital signs
    b. Dehydration
    c. Abdominal girth
    d. Urine for bilirubin

11. The kind of drainage system used for a T tube inserted into the common bile duct after surgery is:
    a. Intermittent suction
    b. Constant low suction
    c. Constant high suction
    d. Closed gravity drainage

12. The action that may provide relief of pain from acute pancreatitis is to:
    a. Give aspirin
    b. Give meperidine (Demerol)
    c. Give morphine
    d. Apply a heating pad to abdomen

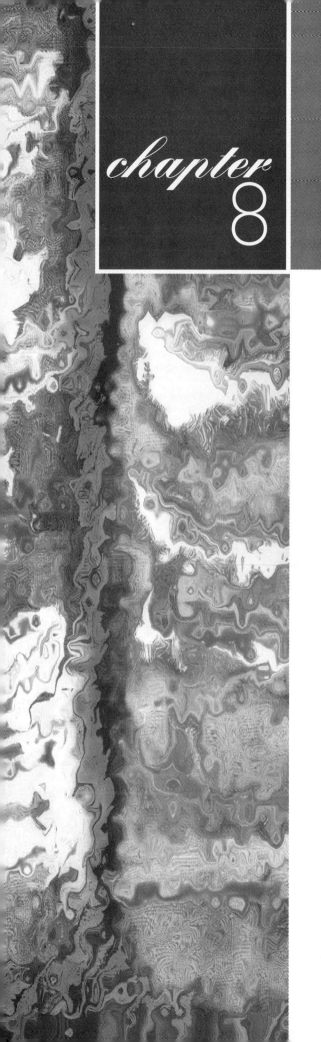

chapter 8

Care of the Patient with a Cardiovascular Disorder

CHAPTER SUMMARY

Chapter 8 describes the anatomy and physiology of the heart and gives a detailed description of how blood circulates through the body. The differences among veins, arteries, and capillaries are detailed. The difference between angina and myocardial infarction (MI) is delineated. The etiology and nursing management of major cardiac and peripheral vascular disorders are presented, along with patient teaching on prevention and risk factors. Also explored are nursing interventions for cardiac patients regarding lifestyle, exercise, and medications.

LEARNING OBJECTIVES

After reading the chapter in the textbook and working through the chapter in this study guide, the student should be able to do the following:

Anatomy and Physiology
- Discuss the location, size, and position of the heart.
- Identify the chambers of the heart.
- List the functions of the chambers of the heart.
- Identify the valves of the heart and their locations.
- Explain what produces the two main heart sounds.
- Discuss the electrical conduction system that causes the cardiac muscle fibers to contract.

Medical-Surgical

- Define the key terms found in the matching exercises.
- Compare nonmodifiable risk factors in coronary artery disease (CAD) with factors that are modifiable in lifestyle and health management.
- List diagnostic tests used to evaluate cardiovascular function.
- Describe five cardiac dysrhythmias.
- Compare etiology/pathophysiology, signs and symptoms, medical management, and nursing interventions for patients with angina pectoris, MI, or congestive heart failure (CHF).
- Specify patient teaching for patients with cardiac dysrhythmias, angina pectoris, MI, CHF, and vascular heart disease.
- List the signs and symptoms of pulmonary edema.
- Discuss nursing interventions for the patient with pulmonary edema.
- Identify risk factors associated with peripheral vascular disorders.
- Describe the effects of aging on the peripheral vascular system.
- Compare and contrast signs and symptoms associated with arterial and venous disorders.
- Discuss nursing interventions for arterial and venous disorders.
- Compare essential (primary) hypertension and secondary hypertension.
- Discuss the importance of patient education for hypertension.
- Discuss appropriate patient education for thrombophlebitis.
- Discuss nursing interventions for the patient with cardiomyopathy.
- Discuss the purpose of cardiac rehabilitation.

KEY TERMS AND DEFINITIONS

_____	1. Angina pectoris
_____	2. Arteriosclerosis
_____	3. Atherosclerosis
_____	4. Congestive heart failure
_____	5. Coronary heart disease
_____	6. Defibrillation
_____	7. Dysrhythmia
_____	8. Embolus
_____	9. Hypoxemia
_____	10. Intermittent claudication
_____	11. Ischemia
_____	12. Myocardial infarction
_____	13. Occlusion
_____	14. Orthopnea
_____	15. Pulmonary edema
_____	16. Tachycardia

a. An occlusion of a major coronary artery or one of its branches with subsequent necrosis of myocardium caused by atherosclerosis or an embolus

b. The termination of ventricular fibrillation by delivering a direct electrical countershock to the patient's precordium

c. An abnormal deficiency of oxygen in the arterial blood

d. The accumulation of extravascular fluid in lung tissue and alveoli, caused mostly by CHF

e. A common arterial disorder characterized by thickening, loss of elasticity, and calcification of arterial walls, resulting in a decreased blood supply

f. A blockage in a canal, vessel, or passage of the body

g. An abnormal condition characterized by circulatory congestion as a result of the heart's inability to act as an effective pump

h. A rapid regular rhythm, originating in the sinoatrial (SA) node

i. Decreased blood supply to a body organ or part, often marked by pain and organ dysfunction

j. Any disturbance or abnormality in a normal cardiac rhythmic pattern

k. An abnormal condition in which a person must sit or stand in order to breath deeply or comfortably

l. A foreign object, a quantity of air or gas, a bit of tissue, or a piece of a thrombus that circulates in the blood stream until it becomes lodged in a vessel

m. A feeling of discomfort in the chest caused by decreased oxygen or anoxia of the myocardium

n. A weakness of the legs accompanied by cramplike pains in the calves caused by poor circulation of the blood to the leg muscles

o. A common arterial disorder characterized by yellowish plaques of cholesterol, lipids, and cellular debris in the inner layers of the walls of large and medium-size arteries

p. The term used to describe a variety of conditions that obstruct blood flow in the coronary arteries

REINFORCING KEY POINTS

1. Explain the purpose of the coronary blood supply.

2. Explain how the heart's electrical conducting system works.

3. Discuss two of the major types of circulation in the body: systemic and pulmonary.

4. Describe the most common signs and symptoms of cardiovascular disease.

5. Describe what information an electrocardiogram (ECG) records.

6. Differentiate between the pain of angina pectoris and MI.

7. Cite the initial signs and symptoms of cardiogenic shock.

8. Discuss the signs and symptoms the nurse will assess as cardiac output decreases.

9. Discuss the etiology and pathophysiology of CHF.

10. Explain why an embolus is so dangerous.

11. Differentiate between a thrombus and an embolus.

12. List the three types of hypertension, and explain how they differ.

APPLICATION OF CLINICAL SKILLS

1. With a diagram of the heart, trace the blood flow through the chambers and valves, labeling the route of circulating blood, beginning and ending in the lungs.

2. Describe the cardiac assessment that would be specific for the older adult, including the changes related to the normal process of aging.

3. Examine an ECG strip, and identify the normal PQRST pattern.

4. Teach a patient about the risk factors associated with hypertension.

5. Demonstrate the sites to which ischemic myocardial pain is most likely to radiate, especially noting the:
   a. Jaw
   b. Chest
   c. Sternum
   d. Left shoulder
   e. Epigastric area

6. Demonstrate how nitroglycerin should be administered, and explain the rationale.

7. Describe the classic signs and symptoms of an MI.

EXERCISES IN FUNDAMENTAL CONCEPTS

1. The main function of the cardiovascular system is that it delivers _____ and _____ to the cells.

2. The upper right chamber, the _____, receives deoxygenated blood from the entire body.

3. The heart has two atrioventricular (AV) valves. They are located between the _____ and _____.

4. The left AV valve is composed of cusps (bicuspid) and is commonly called the _____ _____. It is located between the _____ and _____.

5. The heartbeat is initiated in the _____, which is located in the upper part of the right atrium. Because it regulates the beat of the heart, it is known as the _____.

6. The cardiac cycle refers to a _____.

7. The phase of contraction is called _____, and the phase of relaxation is called _____.

8. There are three main types of blood vessels organized to carry blood to and from the heart: _____ connect the _____ to the _____.

EXERCISES IN CRITICAL THINKING

Topics for Writing

1. Write a nursing care plan emphasizing patient teaching for the patient with CHF.

2. Outline the basic assessment of the cardiovascular system, including these signs and symptoms:
   a. Pain
   b. Cough
   c. Edema
   d. Fatigue
   e. Syncope
   f. Dyspnea
   g. Cyanosis
   h. Orthopnea
   i. Palpitations
   j. Diaphoresis

Topics for Discussion

1. Discuss the emotional impact of an MI on a patient.

2. Discuss the effects that normal aging has on the heart and coronary circulation.

STUDY QUESTIONS

1. The nurse is assessing Mr. Carter, who is exhibiting high levels of anxiety and complaining of chest pain that originates near the sternum. He states the pain is sharp and deep. It is an 8 or 9 on a scale of 10. The next component in the pain assessment should be:
   a. Where the pain is radiating
   b. Where the pain is coming from
   c. Further details of the description
   d. What, if anything, relieves the pain

2. When the cardiac patient complains that his heart is pounding or racing, the nurse should be alert for:
   a. Sudden coughing
   b. Sudden bradycardia
   c. Crackles or wheezing
   d. Dysrhythmia on the ECG

3. The nurse notes that a cardiac patient becomes fatigued and experiences difficulty breathing after getting out of bed and walking to the bathroom. This should be documented as:
   a. Syncope
   b. Muscle ischemia
   c. Fatigue syndrome
   d. Exertional dyspnea

4. The nurse observes that a cardiac patient has difficulty breathing when lying down. This symptom is recognized as:
   a. Syncope
   b. Dyspnea
   c. Orthopnea
   d. Generalized fatigue

5. The nurse is preparing to do patient teaching with Mr. Owens, who has been diagnosed with a cardiovascular disorder. Nonmodifiable factors must be taken into consideration when planning treatment. These factors include:
   a. Smoking
   b. Family history
   c. Dietary control
   d. Hyperlipidemia

6. The diagnostic tests are on the chart of a cardiac patient. In checking these results, it is important to know that the best predictor of the development of a cardiovascular disease is:
   a. Arterial blood gas (ABG) readings
   b. Cholesterol levels
   c. The high-density lipoprotein/low-density lipoprotein (HDL/LDL) ratio
   d. Carbon monoxide levels

7. During patient teaching for the cardiac patient, the nurse describes the myocardium as:
   a. The inner layer of the heart
   b. The outside layer of the heart
   c. The muscular layer of the heart
   d. The fluid between layers of the heart

8. In performing a cardiac assessment the nurse knows that the atrioventricular valves, the tricuspid valve, and the mitral valve are closed:
   a. During systole
   b. During diastole
   c. At all times
   d. When semilunar valves are closed

9. The "lubb-dubb" heart sounds are the first and second sounds heard when auscultating the normal heartbeat. The sounds are caused by:
   a. Blood flowing swiftly through
   b. Tightening of the Purkinje fibers
   c. Reaction of the muscles in the chamber
   d. Closure of the AV nodes and semilunar valves

10. The function of the coronary artery system is:
    a. To balance the heart's circulation
    b. To supply blood to the ventricles
    c. To supply blood to the myocardium
    d. To maintain the stimulus-response process

11. The pacemaker of the heart is the:
    a. Bundle of His
    b. Sinoatrial node
    c. Bachmann's bundle
    d. Atrioventricular node

12. The purpose of a pacemaker is to:
    a. Prevent CHF
    b. Prevent premature ventricular contractions (PVCs)
    c. Regulate heartbeat
    d. Prevent heart attack

13. There are four classifications of lipoproteins in the blood; the "good" lipoproteins are:
    a. RDLs
    b. LDLs
    c. HDLs
    d. VLDLs

14. The stress test takes the patient to the limit of exertion to set the limits of exercise tolerance. This is important to evaluate:
    a. Cardiac disease
    b. Electrical activity
    c. Cardiac capability
    d. Cardiac risk factors

15. The determining factor regarding the seriousness of PVCs and their effect on the heart's ability to pump blood is:
    a. Digitalis toxicity
    b. Location of PVCs
    c. Frequency of PVCs
    d. Medication administered

16. Polycythemia is an abnormal increase of red blood cells in the blood. The cardiac disorder that is associated with polycythemia is:
    a. Sinus tachycardia
    b. Chronic myocarditis
    c. Myocardial infarction
    d. Congestive heart failure

17. The stimulation of red blood cell production by the bone marrow is set off by an abnormal deficiency of oxygen in the arterial blood. This condition is:
    a. Ischemia
    b. Hypoxemia
    c. Hypertension
    d. Hyperlipidemia

18. Angina is differentiated from an MI by which of the following assessments:
    a. Angina pain is always intermittent
    b. Angina begins slowly, MI suddenly
    c. Angina pain goes away, MI pain is persistent
    d. Angina is always accompanied by increased enzymes

19. The physician orders potassium chloride (Slow-K) along with furosemide (Lasix) for the patient who has suffered an MI. The rationale for ordering Slow-K is to:
    a. Dilate vessels
    b. Control edema
    c. Control anxiety
    d. Replace potassium

20. Bed rest is ordered for the patient in danger of cardiogenic shock. The optimal position for this patient is:
    a. Prone
    b. Supine
    c. Lateral
    d. Semi-Fowler's

21. The nurse is taking a history, and the patient states that rheumatic heart disease was diagnosed during childhood. The danger of this disease in later years is:
    a. Chronic pericarditis
    b. MI
    c. Valvular heart disease
    d. CHF

22. While caring for a patient diagnosed with peri-carditis, the nurse is aware that the most danger-ous complication of pericarditis is:
    a. Septic shock
    b. Cardiac arrest
    c. Cardiac tamponade
    d. Ventricular fibrillation

23. The predominant clinical sign of pericarditis is:
    a. Ventricular filling
    b. MI
    c. Pericardial friction rub
    d. Narrowing pulse pressure

24. In treating the patient with an aneurysm, the first priority of care is:
    a. Dissolving clots
    b. Controlling pain
    c. Controlling hypertension
    d. Controlling apprehension

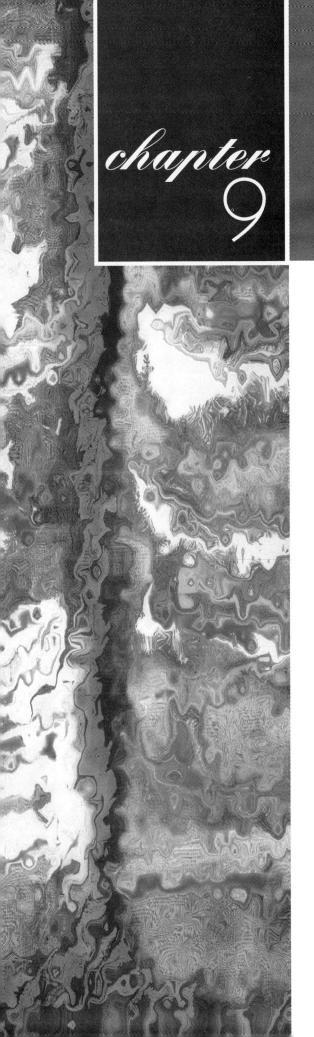

chapter 9

Care of the Patient with a Blood or Lymphatic Disorder

CHAPTER SUMMARY

Chapter 9 presents the anatomy and physiology of the blood and lymphatic system, describing in detail blood components and types as well as the formation of blood. The primary lymphatic structures are described. Much detail is given to the complete blood count and what an elevation or drop in each component could mean. The major disorders associated with the blood and lymphatic systems are presented, with clinical manifestations, medical management, and nursing interventions.

LEARNING OBJECTIVES

After reading the chapter in the textbook and working through the chapter in this study guide, the student should be able to do the following:

Anatomy and Physiology
- Describe the components of blood.
- Differentiate among the functions of erythrocytes, leukocytes, and thrombocytes.
- Discuss the several factors necessary for the formation of erythrocytes.
- Describe what the leukocyte differential means.
- Describe the blood clotting process.
- List the names of the basic blood groups.
- Describe the generalized functions of the lymphatic system, and list the primary lymphatic structures.

Medical-Surgical

- Define the key terms found in the matching exercises.
- List common diagnostic tests for evaluation of blood and lymph disorders, and discuss the significance of the results.
- Apply the nursing process to the care of the patient with disorders of the hematological and lymphatic systems.
- Compare and contrast the different types of anemia in terms of pathophysiology, assessment, and nursing interventions.
- Compare and contrast the disorders of coagulation (thrombocytopenia, hemophilia, disseminated intravascular coagulation [DIC]) in terms of pathophysiology, assessment, and nursing interventions.
- Discuss medical management of patients with hemophilia and DIC.
- List six signs and symptoms associated with hypovolemic shock.
- Discuss important aspects that should be presented in patient teaching and home care planning for the patient with pernicious anemia.
- Discuss the prognosis for patients with acute and chronic leukemia.
- Discuss the primary goal of nursing interventions for the patient with lymphedema.
- Differentiate between Hodgkin's disease and non-Hodgkin's lymphomas and related medical management and nursing interventions.
- Discuss the nursing intervention and patient teaching for the patient with multiple myeloma.

KEY TERMS AND DEFINITIONS

_____	1. Anemia
_____	2. Disseminated intravascular coagulation
_____	3. Erythrocytosis
_____	4. Hemophilia
_____	5. Leukemia
_____	6. Lymphangitis
_____	7. Lymphedema
_____	8. Myeloproliferative
_____	9. Pancytopenic
_____	10. Pernicious
_____	11. Reed-Sternberg cell
_____	12. Thrombocytopenia

a. Excessive bone marrow production
b. A grave coagulopathy resulting from the overstimulation of clotting and anticlotting processes in response to disease or injury, including septicemia, obstetrical complications, malignancies, tissue trauma, transfusion reaction, burns, shock, and snake bites
c. Reduction or absence of all three major blood elements from the bone marrow
d. An abnormal hematological condition in which the number of platelets is reduced
e. A disorder characterized by red blood cell (RBC), hemoglobin, and hematocrit levels below normal range; also exhibits increased RBC destruction
f. An inflammation of one or more lymphatic vessels or channels that usually results from an acute streptococcal or staphylococcal infection in an extremity
g. An abnormal increase in the number of circulating red cells
h. The causing of great injury or destruction; deadly or fatal
i. A malignant disorder of the hematopoietic system in which an excess of leukocytes accumulates in the bone marrow and lymph nodes
j. A hereditary coagulation disorder characterized by a disturbance of the clotting factors
k. Large, abnormal, multinucleated cells in the lymphatic system found in Hodgkin's disease
l. A primary or secondary disorder characterized by the accumulation of lymph in soft tissue and edema

REINFORCING KEY POINTS

1. Describe the components of blood, including pH.

2. Give the normal blood volume in an adult.

3. List the three critical functions of blood.

4. Describe the major functions of the:
   a. Platelets

   b. Red blood cells

   c. White blood cells

5. Describe the steps in the blood clotting process.

6. Cite the four major blood types and how they differ; outline the types that are compatible.

7. Describe signs and symptoms of iron-deficiency anemia.

8. Differentiate among the following anemias, citing the causes and treatments:
   a. Aplastic
   b. Pernicious
   c. Sickle cell
   d. Iron-deficiency

APPLICATION OF CLINICAL SKILLS

1. Provide genetic counseling for a woman whose son has hemophilia.

2. Consider the implications of an 8% eosinophil count in the white blood cell (WBC) differential.

3. Consider the emotional support for a patient who has consented to undergo a bone marrow transplant.

4. Write a care plan emphasizing the dietary requirements for a patient with iron-deficiency anemia.

EXERCISES IN FUNDAMENTAL CONCEPTS

1. Blood is a viscous (thick), red fluid that contains _____, _____, and _____, which are suspended in a light yellow fluid called _____.

2. Blood is slightly _____, with a pH range of 7.35 to 7.45.

3. The blood performs three critical functions. First, it _____ and _____ to the cell and waste products away from the cells. Second, it _____ with buffers, aids with body temperature because of its water content, and controls the water content as a result of dissolved sodium ions. Third, it _____ with special cells and prevents blood loss with special clotting mechanisms.

4. _____ give blood its rich color.

5. The average life span of an RBC is _____.

6. WBCs are called _____ and respond predictably to symptoms of infection.

7. A differential white blood cell count is _____ _____.

8. Platelets are called _____ and function in the _____.

9. A person's blood group or type is determined _____ and _____.

10. _____ can be used in an emergency as donor blood without the danger of anti-A or anti-B antibodies clumping its RBCs and is called universal donor blood.

11. _____ has been called the universal recipient blood because it contains neither anti-A nor anti-B antibodies in its plasma.

EXERCISES IN CRITICAL THINKING

Topics for Writing

1. Describe the feedback mechanism that controls the rate at which RBCs are made.

2. List the five WBCs and what significance an increase or decrease in each might have.

Topics for Discussion

1. Discuss the meaning of a shift to the left and what pathological process it indicates.

2. Discuss the difference between bleeding time and clotting time and the implications of each.

3. Discuss the importance of and implications related to the immune system of the following lymphatic structures:
   a. Tonsils
   b. Spleen
   c. Thymus

STUDY QUESTIONS

1. The blood has a pH range of 7.35 to 7.45. This means that the blood is slightly:
   a. Salty
   b. Acidic
   c. Plasma
   d. Alkaline

2. The blood type known as the universal donor is:
   a. A
   b. B
   c. O
   d. AB

3. The substance in the blood that carries oxygen to the cells and carbon dioxide away from the cells is:
   a. Hematocrit
   b. Erythrocytes
   c. Hemoglobin
   d. Reticulocytes

4. Mr. Johnson is hospitalized after multiple injuries in a car accident. On the third day following admission, the nurse assesses purpura on the chest and abdomen. The nurse immediately calls the physician because:
   a. This is an early sign of DIC
   b. Mr. Johnson may be bleeding internally
   c. Mr. Johnson may need emergency surgery
   d. Mr. Johnson may need a blood transfusion

5. The physician has ordered a Schilling test, and it is positive. This is the diagnostic test for:
   a. Aplastic anemia
   b. Pernicious anemia
   c. Folic acid deficiency
   d. Iron-deficiency anemia

6. Mrs. Newton has been admitted to the hospital complaining of enlarged, although painless lymph nodes, fever, weight loss, and pruritus. Diagnostic tests have been ordered related to:
   a. Thrombocytopenia
   b. Hodgkin's disease
   c. Malignant myeloma
   d. Malignant lymphoma

7. The Rh-negative mother is protected from future Rh incompatibility:
   a. With IV RhoGAM
   b. With an IM injection of RhoGAM
   c. By her body naturally making antigens
   d. By her body naturally building antibodies

8. In planning care for the patient with anemia, the major clinical consideration is:
   a. The urge to binge
   b. Depressed mood
   c. Danger of hemorrhage
   d. Insufficient O2 to cells

9. The medication most likely to be prescribed for the patient who has had a bone marrow transplant is:
   a. Cephalexin (Keflex)
   b. Penicillin
   c. Vitamin K
   d. Cyclosporine

10. The nurse is assessing blood loss in a patient who is threatened with hypovolemic shock. The signs most closely monitored are:
    a. Hypotension, bradycardia
    b. Hypotension, tachycardia
    c. Hypertension, tachycardia
    d. Decreased respiration, pulse

11. The nurse should instruct the patient who has been diagnosed with pernicious anemia that B_{12} injections will be prescribed once every month for:
    a. 1 year
    b. 2 years
    c. Life
    d. 6 months

12. In assessing a new patient, which of the following data is most indicative of a blood disorder?
    a. Sunken eyes and pallor
    b. Complaints of restlessness
    c. Fatigue and easy bruising
    d. Depression and mood swings

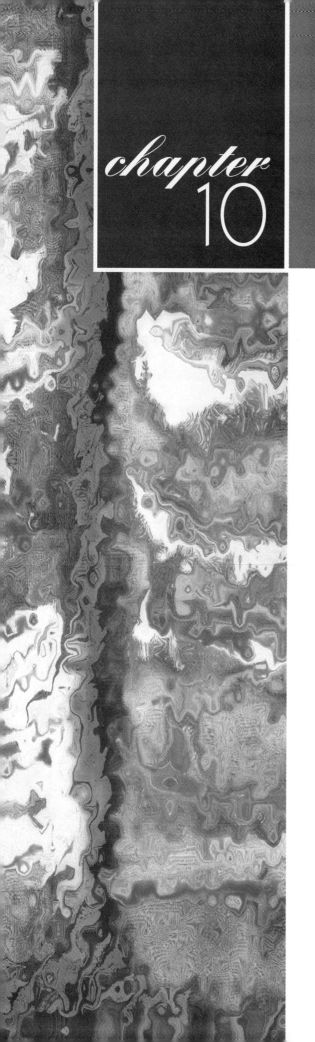

chapter 10

Care of the Patient with a Urinary Disorder

CHAPTER SUMMARY

Chapter 10 reviews the anatomical structures of the urinary system and gives a detailed physiological description of how they work. The influence of hormones on nephron functioning is considered. Based on an understanding of normal functioning, urinary problems and dysfunction are discussed, and the nursing diagnoses are listed along with the priorities and special needs of the patient with urinary dysfunction. The nurse's role in dialysis and other renal problems is also detailed in nursing care plans. Pharmacotherapeutic and nutritional considerations for urinary disorders are emphasized.

LEARNING OBJECTIVES

After reading the chapter in the textbook and working through the chapter in this study guide, the student should be able to do the following:

Anatomy and Physiology
- Describe the structures of the urinary system, including functions.
- List the three processes involved in urine formation.
- Discuss the normal versus abnormal components of urine.
- Name three hormones and their influence on nephron function.

Medical-Surgical

- Define the key terms found in the matching exercises.
- Describe the alterations in renal function associated with disorders of the urinary tract.
- Select nursing diagnoses related to alterations in urinary function.
- Prioritize the special needs of the patient with urinary dysfunction.
- Appraise the changes in body image created when the patient experiences an alteration in urinary function.
- Identify the effects of aging on urinary system function.
- Adapt teaching methods for the patient with urinary disorders.
- Discuss the impact of renal disease on family function.
- Incorporate pharmacotherapeutic and nutritional considerations into the nursing care plan of the patient with a urinary disorder.

KEY TERMS AND DEFINITIONS

_____	1. Anasarca
_____	2. Anuria
_____	3. Azotemia
_____	4. Bacteriuria
_____	5. Dysuria
_____	6. Ileal conduit
_____	7. Nocturia
_____	8. Oliguria
_____	9. Pyuria
_____	10. Residual urine
_____	11. Retention
_____	12. Urolithiasis

a. Excessive urination at night
b. Severe generalized edema
c. The retention of excessive amounts of nitrogenous compounds in the blood
d. Painful urination
e. Urinary stones
f. Pus in the urine
g. Presence of bacteria in the urine
h. A diminished capacity to form and pass urine
i. Urinary output less than 100 ml/day
j. The inability to void even when an urge to void is present
k. Procedure where the ureters are implanted into a loop of the ileum that is isolated and brought to the surface of the abdominal wall
l. The amount of urine retained in the bladder

REINFORCING KEY POINTS

1. Describe the location of the kidneys.

2. Describe the functioning unit of the kidney.

3. Cite the three phases of urine formation.

4. Define the word _hematuria_, and explain its significance.

5. Explain what leukocytes in the urine indicate.

6. Outline the information that should be gathered when taking a nursing assessment of urinary function.

7. Discuss the information that can be gathered with a routine urinalysis.

8. Cite the purpose of measuring the blood urea nitrogen (BUN) and the creatinine clearance values.

9. Discuss for what purposes a kidney, ureter, and bladder (KUB) x-ray and an intravenous pyelogram (IVP) are ordered.

10. Describe cystoscopy, and the purpose for which it is done.

11. Cite the nursing interventions required after a renal biopsy.

12. Discuss the action of diuretics.

13. Differentiate among the following diuretics, and give an example of each:
    a. Thiazides

    b. Loop diuretics

    c. Osmotic diuretics

    d. Potassium-sparing diuretics

14. Discuss the actions of Urecholine.

15. Cite the actions of the following medications prescribed for urinary tract infections:
    a. Methenamine mandelate (Mandelamine)

    b. Norfloxacin (Noroxin)

    c. Nalidixic acid (NegGram)

    d. Nitrofurantoin (Macrodantin)

16. Describe the different kinds of catheters, including the Foley.

17. Cite nursing interventions required for the patient with a catheter.

18. Define urinary retention and residual urine, and discuss the significance of each.

19. Discuss the problem of urinary incontinence and when it is most likely to occur.

20. Cite the pathophysiology and medical management for:
    a. Cystitis

    b. Urethritis

    c. Prostatitis

    d. Urolithiasis

    e. Pyelonephritis

    f. Urinary tract infections

21. Outline the nursing interventions that are important when a patient is experiencing urolithiasis (urinary stones).

22. Define benign prostatic hypertrophy (BPH).

23. List the four types of surgery that may be performed for BPH.

24. Discuss the nursing interventions for BPH and for transurethral prostatic resection (TURP).

25. Cite the clinical manifestations of nephrotic syndrome.

26. Differentiate between acute and chronic glomerulonephritis.

27. Review the guidelines for the patient undergoing hemodialysis.

28. Identify the distal convoluted tubule, collecting tubules, proximal convoluted tubule, and the thin segment of Henle's loop in the figure below:

APPLICATION OF CLINICAL SKILLS

1. Describe the procedure for catheterizing a female patient.

2. Describe the procedure for catheterizing a male patient.

3. Describe the procedure for catheter care for a female patient and a male patient.

4. Describe the procedure for catheter irrigation.

5. Describe the procedure for discontinuing a Foley catheter.

6. Describe the procedure for bladder instillation.

7. Cite nursing interventions for the patient in renal failure.

8. Explain why catheterization is a sterile procedure.

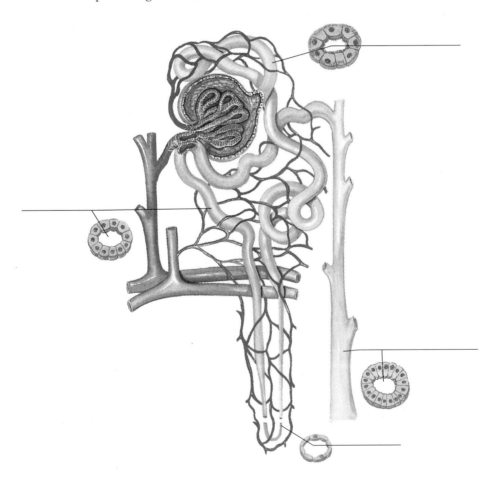

9. Document the results after inserting a Foley catheter, including a description of the urine.

10. Outline the teaching required for the patient who has a catheter.

11. Instruct a patient on strengthening pelvic muscles to stop stress incontinence.

12. Teach the patient with nephrotic syndrome about a high-protein, low-sodium diet.

EXERCISES IN FUNDAMENTAL CONCEPTS

1. The urinary system is probably the most important system in _____.

2. Because of the size and shape of the liver, the _____ kidney lies slightly lower than the left.

3. The _____ is the functional unit of the kidney, and each kidney contains more than _____ nephrons. Its function is to _____ and _____.

4. _____, or hydrostatic pressure, determines the glomerular filtration rate (GFR).

5. The body forms _____ to _____ of urine per day.

6. Urine is _____ with a pH of _____ to _____.

7. When the bladder contains approximately _____ of urine, the individual has a conscious desire to urinate.

8. A moderately full bladder holds _____ (1 pint) of urine.

EXERCISES IN CRITICAL THINKING

Topics for Writing

1. Outline the filtration of water through the kidneys, particularly mentioning each major structure.

2. List the major functions of the kidneys and their implications for overall body functioning.

Topics for Discussion

1. Discuss the gerontological considerations for the patient who has a urinary or renal disorder.

2. Discuss why it is so difficult for a patient with cystitis to be cured of the disorder.

3. Discuss the different ways that urinary incontinence can be alleviated.

STUDY QUESTIONS

1. A culture and sensitivity urine test has been ordered for a patient with urinary symptoms. This test is done to detect:
   a. Diabetes mellitus
   b. Kidney obstruction
   c. Causative organisms
   d. Extent of kidney disease

2. Mrs. Carter is scheduled for a BUN test. The nurse must keep Mrs. Carter NPO for:
   a. 2 hours
   b. 8 hours
   c. 10 hours
   d. 12 hours

3. Mr. Bates is scheduled for a creatinine clearance test. Patient teaching should include:
   a. Avoid excessive physical activity
   b. Drink plenty of water on the day before the test
   c. Do not eat protein 24 hours before the test
   d. Do not eat for the 24-hour testing period

4. Mr. Stevens is scheduled for an IVP to evaluate structures of the urinary tract. It is vital that the nurse chart:
   a. Blood pressure
   b. Allergy to iodine
   c. Recent food intake
   d. Elevated temperature

5. Mr. Anson is preparing for a magnetic resonance imaging (MRI). The nurse is aware that there is no special preparation for a MRI. The only precaution that must be taken is:
   a. NPO for 12 hours
   b. Electrocardiogram (ECG) must be on chart
   c. All metal objects must be removed
   d. Antianxiety medication must be ordered

6. Mrs. Bates is to undergo a needle biopsy of the kidney. This is a painful procedure. Patient education for this procedure is specific and must include:
   a. NPO for 24 hours
   b. Holding breath during procedure
   c. No physical activity before procedure
   d. Take pain medication before procedure

7. Serum creatinine and BUN are tests that measure:
   a. Ability to eliminate dye
   b. Ability to conserve body fluid
   c. Ability to eliminate metabolic wastes
   d. Regulation of electrolyte concentration

8. The kind of urine specimen required for a creatinine clearance test is:
   a. Clean catch
   b. 24-hour urine
   c. Sterile specimen
   d. Early-morning urine

9. During a timed urine specimen collection, the first and last specimens collected should:
   a. Both be discarded
   b. Both be sent to the laboratory
   c. First specimen discarded, last specimen sent to the laboratory
   d. First specimen sent to the laboratory, last specimen discarded

10. The procedure required before an intravenous urogram (IVU) is done is:
    a. NPO
    b. KUB
    c. Electroencephalogram (EEG)
    d. ECG

11. When interviewing a female patient with a urinary disorder, the nurse must be aware that one of the symptoms of urinary tract infection is:
    a. Anuria
    b. Dysuria
    c. Polyuria
    d. Nocturia

12. The nurse is preparing a teaching plan for a patient with urinary tract infection; teaching must include the following information or advice:
    a. Recurrences are infrequent
    b. Increase fluid intake to 2000 ml/day
    c. Eat foods that maintain alkaline urine
    d. Medication is discontinued when symptoms abate

13. The nurse suspects obstruction of the upper urinary tract with backflow. The condition requires priority because it can lead to:
    a. Renal calculi
    b. Hydronephrosis
    c. Polycystic kidney
    d. Urinary incontinence

14. A newly admitted patient is suspected of having urinary stones. In assessing this patient the nurse is aware that the hallmark of urinary stones is:
    a. Distention
    b. Hematuria
    c. Severe pain
    d. Hypertension

15. The nurse is assessing a male with a history of BPH. The clinical picture of BPH is basically:
    a. Cancer of the prostate
    b. Location of the prostate
    c. Enlargement of the prostate
    d. Loss of function of the prostate

16. During the interview with a patient who has BPH the nurse recognizes that the earliest symptom is:
    a. Dysuria
    b. Nocturia
    c. Hematuria
    d. Frequency

17. The patient who has been diagnosed with acute pyelonephritis is suspected now to have the chronic condition. The difference between acute and chronic pyelonephritis is:
    a. Malaise, flank pain
    b. Positive urine culture
    c. Fever, flank tenderness
    d. Duration of inflammation

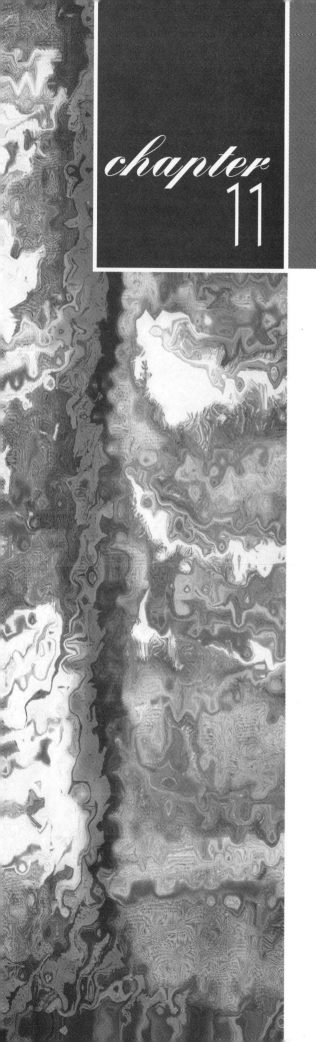

chapter 11

Care of the Patient with a Respiratory Disorder

CHAPTER SUMMARY

Chapter 11 reviews the anatomy and physiology of the upper and lower respiratory systems and the mechanisms that regulate respiration and the exchange of oxygen and carbon dioxide. Nursing interventions are presented for several conditions, including hypoxia, pneumonia, tuberculosis, chronic obstructive pulmonary disease (COPD), laryngectomy, and pulmonary embolism. Nursing assessments and interventions pertaining to the care of the patient with chest tubes are discussed. The important psychosocial concerns of respiratory patients are also addressed.

LEARNING OBJECTIVES

After reading the chapter in the textbook and working through the chapter in this study guide, the student should be able to do the following:

Anatomy and Physiology
- List and define the parts of the upper and lower respiratory tracts.
- Describe the purpose of the respiratory system.
- Differentiate between external and internal respiration.
- List the ways in which oxygen and carbon dioxide are transported in the blood.
- Discuss the mechanisms that regulate respirations.

Medical-Surgical

- Define the key terms found in the matching exercises.
- List five nursing interventions to assist patients with retained pulmonary secretions.
- Identify signs and symptoms that indicate a patient is experiencing hypoxia.
- Identify four strategies the nurse can teach patients to decrease risk of infection.
- Differentiate between tuberculosis infection and tuberculosis disease.
- List three medications commonly prescribed for the patient with tuberculosis.
- Differentiate between medical management of the patient with emphysema and the patient with asthma.
- Discuss why low-flow oxygen is required for patients with emphysema.
- Compare and contrast nursing assessment and interventions for the patient with COPD and the patient with pneumonia.
- List three nursing assessments or interventions pertaining to the care of the patient with closed chest drainage.
- Discuss nursing interventions for the patient with a laryngectomy.
- State three possible nursing diagnoses for the patient with altered respiratory function.
- Identify nursing interventions relevant to psychosocial concerns of the patient with altered respiratory function.
- Discuss three risk factors associated with pulmonary emboli.

KEY TERMS AND DEFINITIONS

_____ 1. Adventitious
_____ 2. Atelectasis
_____ 3. Bronchoscopy
_____ 4. Crackles
_____ 5. Epistaxis
_____ 6. Hemoptysis
_____ 7. Hypercapnia
_____ 8. Hypoventilation
_____ 9. Hypoxia
_____ 10. Orthopnea
_____ 11. Pleural friction rub
_____ 12. Pneumothorax
_____ 13. Sibilant wheezes
_____ 14. Sonorous wheezes
_____ 15. Stertorous
_____ 16. Tachypnea
_____ 17. Thoracentesis

a. Abnormal rate of breathing; more than 26 breaths/min
b. A collection of air or gas in the pleural cavity causing the lung to collapse
c. Abnormal condition characterized by cyanosis, clubbing of the fingers, Cheyne-Stokes breathing, and generally decreased respiratory function
d. Breathing characterized by a bubbling or whistling sound upon inspiration
e. The surgical perforation of the chest wall
f. An abnormal condition characterized by the collapse of lung tissues preventing the respiratory exchange of carbon dioxide and oxygen
g. Expectorating blood from the respiratory tract
h. Abnormal condition in which person must sit or stand to breathe
i. Abnormal breath sounds arising sporadically or in other than their usual location
j. Excessive amounts of carbon dioxide in the blood
k. Visual examination of the tracheobronchial tree, using the standard metal bronchoscope or the narrower, flexible fiberoptic bronchoscope
l. Breathing characterized by a harsh snoring or gasping sound
m. Bleeding from the nose
n. Low-pitched, grating, or creaking lung sounds that occur when inflamed pleural surfaces rub together during respirations
o. Musical sounds that are created when air is forced through respiratory passages narrowed by fluid, mucus, or pus
p. Inadequate amount of oxygen available at the cellular level, characterized by cyanosis, tachycardia, hypertension, peripheral vasoconstriction, vertigo, and mental confusion
q. Breathing characterized by low-pitched, loud, coarse, snoring sounds

REINFORCING KEY POINTS

1. Differentiate between internal and external respiration.

2. Describe how respiration takes place in the lungs and what happens during this process.

3. Define pleural effusion, and explain its significance.

4. Name the parts of the brain that control respiration.

5. Explain how carbon dioxide stimulates respiration.

6. Discuss the data that the respiratory assessment includes.

7. The nurse documents "orthopnea"; explain what this means.

8. Briefly define each of the following diagnostic tests, noting the purpose of each and the preparation required by each test:
   a. Chest x-ray

   b. Thoracentesis

   c. Bronchoscopy

   d. Laryngoscopy

   e. Computed tomography (CT) scan of lung

   f. Mediastinoscopy

   g. Cytology studies

   h. Sputum specimen

   i. Arterial blood gases

   j. Pulmonary function testing

9. Note the nursing interventions for patients with:
   a. Epistaxis

   b. Deviated septum

   c. Upper airway obstruction

10. Name the first symptom of cancer of the larynx.

11. Explain why nasopharyngeal suctioning and endotracheal suctioning are sterile procedures.

12. Note the interventions necessary in caring for a tracheostomy collar, or T-piece.

APPLICATION OF CLINICAL SKILLS

1. Describe the signs and symptoms of hypoxia.

2. Describe the procedure for sputum collection.

3. Differentiate between pharyngitis and sinusitis.

4. Explain medications required for the patient with tuberculosis.

5. Explain the medical management and nursing interventions required for the patient with pneumonia.

6. Describe the nursing assessment crucial when monitoring for pulmonary embolus.

7. Cite medical management and nursing interventions for the patient with adult respiratory distress syndrome (ARDS).

8. Explain the purpose of a nebulizer treatment.

9. Perform postural drainage, explaining the purpose and the positions.

10. Demonstrate the administration of oxygen via nasal cannula and by mask.

EXERCISES IN FUNDAMENTAL CONCEPTS

1. The pharynx, or _____, is the passageway for both _____ and _____.

2. Because the inner lining of the _____ and the _____ are continuous, an infection of the pharynx can spread easily to the ear.

3. _____ are small, hair-like processes on the outer surfaces of small cells, aiding metabolism by producing motion or current in a fluid.

4. When a patient has a tracheostomy he or she cannot speak because _____.

5. When a foreign object is aspirated, it is most likely to enter the _____.

6. Gas exchange of _____ and _____ by the process of _____ takes place in a single grapelike structure called an _____.

7. The normal range of respirations for an adult is _____ to _____ respirations/min.

8. Specialized receptors that are sensitive to carbon dioxide and oxygen levels in the blood and can modify respiratory rates are called _____.

9. _____ is the chemical stimulant for the regulation of respiration. Therefore, when the blood becomes acidic, respirations _____.

10. Difficulty breathing, or _____, is a subjective experience that the patient describes.

11. _____ is an abnormal condition in which a person must sit or stand in order to breathe deeply or comfortably.

12. The presence of _____ sounds indicates abnormal breath sounds.

13. Identify the following breath sounds:
    a. Musical, high-pitched
       _____
    b. Low-pitched, loud, coarse
       _____
    c. Short, discrete, bubbling
       _____
    d. Low-pitched, grating
       _____

14. The illustration below shows a complete collapse of the right lung called a _____.

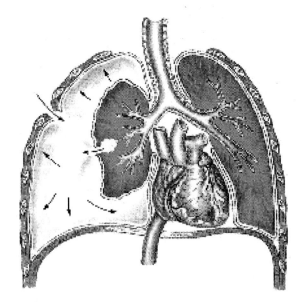

EXERCISES IN CRITICAL THINKING

Topics for Writing

1. Outline the formula or guidelines for interpretation of arterial blood gases (ABGs).

2. Write a patient teaching plan, including diagnosis, tests, and medical management for patients with:
   a. Asthma
   b. Emphysema
   c. Cystic fibrosis
   d. Chronic bronchitis

Topics for Discussion

1. Discuss how the nurse can provide emotional support to the patient with chronic respiratory problems.

2. Differentiate among the following respiratory infections, including signs and symptoms and nursing interventions:
   a. Sinusitis
   b. Bronchitis
   c. Tonsillitis
   d. Laryngitis
   e. Pharyngitis
   f. Common cold

STUDY QUESTIONS

1. The patient is scheduled for a thoracentesis. The nurse instructs the patient that the needle will be inserted into the:
   a. Lungs
   b. Thorax
   c. Bronchi
   d. Pleural space

2. In preparing for a thoracentesis the nurse instructs the patient that the optimal position while undergoing a thoracentesis is:
   a. Prone with hands over head
   b. Supine with hands over head
   c. Lying on unaffected side, with hands over head
   d. Sitting up on side of bed, leaning on overbed table

3. The mother of an 8-year-old boy tells the nurse that her son's nose bleeds "almost every day." The nurse tells her that the most common cause of nosebleed is:
   a. Trauma
   b. Infection
   c. Picking at nose
   d. Lack of humidity

4. An early symptom of cancer of the larynx is:
   a. Hoarseness
   b. Sore throat
   c. Swelling of neck
   d. Enlarged lymph nodes of neck

5. The final effect on breathing after a total laryngectomy is:
   a. Normal breathing
   b. Labored breathing through the nose
   c. Through a temporary tracheostomy
   d. Through a permanent tracheostomy

6. The common name for acute coryza is:
   a. Sinus
   b. Hay fever
   c. Nosebleed
   d. Common cold

7. The disease that causes acute pharyngitis and is becoming increasingly common is:
   a. Syphilis
   b. Herpes
   c. Tonsillitis
   d. Gonorrhea

8. A significant positive reaction in a tuberculin skin test is:
   a. Redness
   b. Severe rash
   c. Skin reaction
   d. An area of hardened tissue

9. The test necessary for a definitive diagnosis of tuberculosis is:
   a. Sputum culture
   b. Chest x-ray film
   c. Positive Mantoux test
   d. Positive tuberculin skin test

10. The sputum collection most productive of organisms is:
    a. After meals
    b. Before meals
    c. First one in morning
    d. Last one before retiring at night

11. The term used to document pus in the pleural space is:
    a. Pleurisy
    b. Empyema
    c. Emphysema
    d. Pleural effusion

12. The condition in which there is an accumulation of secretions resulting in collapsed portions of the lungs is:
    a. Atelectasis
    b. Hemothorax
    c. Pneumothorax
    d. Pleural effusion

13. The cause of lung collapse with pneumothorax is:
    a. Increased fluid pressure
    b. Decreased alveolar pressure
    c. Negative intrapleural pressure
    d. Interrupting the normal negative pressure

14. The pulmonary disorder in which consolidation of alveolar space from filling by exudates occurs is:
    a. Cancer
    b. Bronchitis
    c. Pneumonia
    d. Emphysema

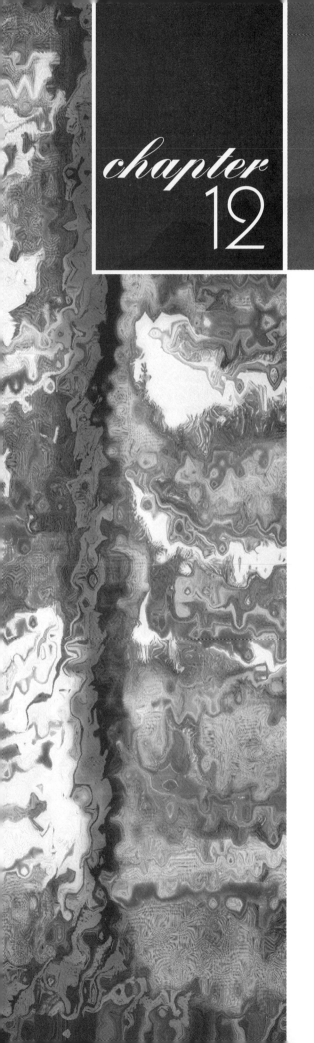

chapter 12

Care of the Patient with an Endocrine Disorder

CHAPTER SUMMARY

Chapter 12 describes the endocrine system, including how hormones work in a negative feedback system. The actions of hormones on their target organs are detailed, in particular how the hypothalamus is involved in hormonal activity. Disorders of the endocrine system are discussed with emphasis on nursing assessment and interventions. Additional emphasis is given to diabetes mellitus, the administration of insulin, and the signs of complications in patients with diabetes; and, finally, the focus is placed on self-care of the patient with diabetes.

LEARNING OBJECTIVES

After reading the chapter in the textbook and working through the chapter in this study guide, the student should be able to do the following:

Anatomy and Physiology

- Define the key terms found in the matching exercises.
- List and describe the endocrine glands and their hormones.
- Explain the action of the hormones on their target organs.
- Define the negative feedback system.
- Describe how the hypothalamus controls the anterior and posterior pituitary glands.

Medical-Surgical

- Define the key terms found in the matching exercises.
- List four clinical manifestations of diabetes insipidus.
- List three tests used in the diagnosis of hyperthyroidism.
- Give the clinical manifestations for patients with acromegaly, gigantism, pheochromocytoma, and hypoparathyroidism.
- Explain how to test for Chvostek's sign and Trousseau's sign.
- List two significant complications that may occur after thyroidectomy.
- Differentiate between clinical manifestations of Cushing's syndrome and those of Addison's disease.
- Explain the interrelationship of diet, exercise, and medication in the control of diabetes mellitus.
- Describe the proper way to draw up and administer insulin.
- Differentiate between the signs and symptoms of diabetic ketoacidosis (DKA), hyperglycemic hyperosmolar nonketotic coma (HHNC), and hypoglycemic reaction.
- List four nursing interventions that foster self-care in the activities of daily living of the patient with diabetes mellitus.

KEY TERMS AND DEFINITIONS

_____	1. Dysphagia
_____	2. Glycosuria
_____	3. Hyperglycemia
_____	4. Hypocalcemia
_____	5. Hypoglycemia
_____	6. Hypokalemia
_____	7. Ketoacidosis
_____	8. Neuropathy
_____	9. Polydipsia
_____	10. Polyphagia
_____	11. Polyuria
_____	12. Type I diabetes mellitus

a. Excessive hunger
b. Insulin-dependent diabetes; formerly called juvenile diabetes or juvenile-onset diabetes
c. Any abnormal condition characterized by inflammation and degeneration of the peripheral nerves
d. Abnormally low level of potassium in the blood
e. Abnormally high level of glucose in the blood

f. Abnormal accumulation of ketones in the body, resulting from faulty carbohydrate metabolism, occurring primarily as a complication of diabetes mellitus
g. Difficulty in swallowing, commonly associated with obstructive or motor disorders of the esophagus
h. Excretion of abnormally large amounts of urine
i. Excessive thirst
j. Abnormally low level of glucose in the blood
k. Abnormal presence of sugar, especially glucose in the urine
l. Abnormally low level of calcium in the blood

REINFORCING KEY POINTS

1. Describe how hormones have a generalized impact on body functions.

2. Explain how the negative feedback system works in regard to hormone functioning.

3. Describe the pituitary hormones and name their target organs.

4. Identify which gland is called the master gland, and explain why.

5. The hormones have dramatic effects on the body; state the functions of these important hormones:
   a. Prolactin

   b. Luteinizing hormone (LH)

   c. Human growth hormone (HGH)

   d. Follicle-stimulating hormone (FSH)

e. Thyroid-stimulating hormone (TSH)

f. Adrenocorticotropic hormone (ACTH)

6. List the three functions of the thyroid hormones.

7. Name the two minerals that are controlled by the parathyroid gland.

8. Explain how aldosterone, secreted by the adrenal cortex, regulates the fluid and electrolyte balance in the body.

9. Name the hormones released by the adrenal medulla, especially in times of stress.

10. Describe the actions the sex hormones, estrogen and progesterone, have on the body.

11. Explain what causes the signs and symptoms of diabetes insipidus.

12. List the three complications the nurse must be alert for after a thyroidectomy.

13. Name the electrolyte imbalance that is usually present in Cushing's syndrome.

14. Define Addison's disease, and list the signs and symptoms.

15. Differentiate between diabetes mellitus types I and II concerning:
a. Weight

b. Symptoms

c. Treatment

d. Age of onset

e. Complications

16. List the cardinal signs and symptoms of non-insulin-dependent diabetes mellitus (NIDDM).

17. Describe the six diagnostic tests that are used to diagnose diabetes mellitus.

18. List the signs and symptoms of a hypoglycemic reaction.

19. Identify the endocrine glands in the figure below:

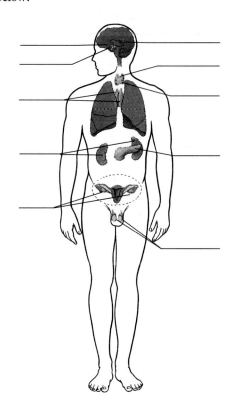

APPLICATION OF CLINICAL SKILLS

1. Write a patient teaching plan for the person with NIDDM.

2. Instruct a patient on the initial signs and symptoms of diabetes mellitus.

3. Instruct a patient on monitoring for onset and peak action of regular and neutral protamine Hagedorn (NPH) insulins.

4. Teach a diabetic patient the signs and symptoms of diabetic ketoacidosis and a hypoglycemic reaction.

5. Demonstrate Chvostek's sign, and explain the significance of a positive sign.

6. Demonstrate Trousseau's sign, and explain the significance of a positive sign.

7. Teach an insulin-dependent patient how to give an insulin injection.

8. Teach a patient to do a finger stick to test blood glucose.

EXERCISES IN FUNDAMENTAL CONCEPTS

1. The two broad categories of glands are _____ and _____. _____ secrete through a series of ducts, such as sebaceous and sudoriferous glands of the skin. Their secretions are protective and functional. _____ are ductless; they release their secretions directly into the blood stream. Their secretions have a regulatory function.

2. _____ are chemical messengers that travel through the blood stream to their target organ.

3. The amount of hormonal release is controlled by a _____ system, which is a decrease in function in response to stimuli.

4. The pituitary gland is called the master gland because _____.

5. ADH causes the kidneys to conserve water by _____. ADH is sometimes called vasopressin because _____.

6. Adequate intake of _____ is necessary for the formation of thyroid hormones.

7. When calcium levels are low, the nerve cells become excited and stimulate the muscles with many impulses, resulting in _____.

8. The two hormones that are released during times of stress are _____ or _____ and _____. They can cause the heart rate and blood pressure to increase, the blood vessels to contract, and the liver to release glucose reserves for immediate energy. This is a systemic preparation of the body for the _____ that is needed in times of crisis.

9. The islets of Langerhans of the _____ secrete two major hormones: _____ and _____.

10. The two hormones that the ovaries produce are _____ and _____. These hormones are responsible for _____ and _____.

11. The testes release the hormone _____, which is responsible for the development of the male secondary sex characteristics.

12. The thymus gland plays an active role in the _____.

13. The pineal gland secretes the hormone _____, which is thought to induce sleep and may also affect one's mood.

EXERCISES IN CRITICAL THINKING

Topics for Writing

1. List the major factors that differentiate type I and type II diabetes mellitus.

2. Sketch a picture of the body, noting where to rotate injection sites for insulin.

Topics for Discussion

1. Discuss the negative feedback system that controls the release of hormones throughout the body.

2. Discuss why the pituitary gland is called the master gland, and describe how it interconnects to the brain.

3. Discuss how diet, exercise, and medication work together to control diabetes mellitus.

4. Discuss the differences between oral hypoglycemics and the administration of insulin.

5. Describe emergency care for the patient with DKA, including the first priorities that the nurse must take.

STUDY QUESTIONS

1. Five hormones are involved in the regulation of blood. The one that lowers the blood glucose is:
   a. Insulin
   b. Glucagon
   c. Epinephrine
   d. Glucocorticoids

2. A distinguishing feature of the endocrine system under which many hormones function is:
   a. The thyroid gland
   b. The hypothalamus
   c. Negative feedback
   d. Regulatory functions

3. The two hormones actually produced in the hypothalamus are:
   a. ADH and oxytocin
   b. Aldosterone and ACTH
   c. Estrogen and testosterone
   d. Growth hormone and ACTH

4. Sodium, potassium, and water in the body are regulated mainly by this group of hormones:
   a. Glucocorticoids
   b. Growth hormones
   c. Hydroxycorticoids
   d. Mineralocorticoids

5. Epinephrine and norepinephrine are secreted by the:
   a. Thyroid
   b. Thymus
   c. Hypothalamus
   d. Adrenal medulla

6. The target organ for growth hormone (GH) is the:
   a. Gonads
   b. Pituitary
   c. Whole body
   d. Adrenal cortex

7. Mr. Owens has a decreased secretion of antidiuretic hormone (ADH) from the posterior pituitary gland. His diagnosis is:
   a. Dwarfism
   b. Myxedema
   c. Acromegaly
   d. Diabetes insipidus

8. Hyperthyroidism's primary effect is:
   a. Increased metabolic rate
   b. Increased calcium metabolism
   c. Overproduction of triiodothyronine
   d. Accumulation of hydrophilic mucopolysaccharides

9. Mrs. Stevens has been diagnosed with the disorder of hyperthyroidism. This is called:
   a. Burn's disorder
   b. Down's disease
   c. Graves' disease
   d. Gordon's disease

10. Mrs. Dennis has been diagnosed with a goiter. She asks what caused it to grow. The nurse tells her that the major cause of goiter is:
    a. Iodine deficiency
    b. Radioactive iodine therapy
    c. Inflammation of the thyroid gland
    d. Surgical removal of the parathyroid gland

11. Mr. Parker is in much pain and is admitted to the hospital. He is diagnosed with a low functioning parathyroid. A characteristic symptom of hypoparathyroidism is:
    a. Tetany
    b. Polyuria
    c. Bone pain
    d. Renal stones

12. The following characteristic would be found in relationship to insulin-dependent diabetes mellitus (IDDM):
    a. Is generally resistant to ketosis
    b. Usually occurs in persons younger than 30 years
    c. Is often called maturity-onset diabetes
    d. Occurs in the majority of persons with diabetes

13. Mrs. Stone, 44 years old, is experiencing the classic signs and symptoms of type II diabetes. One of the three classic signs of hyperglycemia is polyuria, which means:
    a. Increased thirst
    b. Increased appetite
    c. Increased urine output
    d. Increased craving for sweets

14. A common complication of lower extremities seen in persons with diabetes mellitus is:
    a. Keloid
    b. Ulcerations
    c. Varicose veins
    d. Thrombophlebitis

15. The initial signs and symptoms of type II diabetes are:
    a. Increased metabolic production
    b. Polyuria, polydipsia, polyphagia
    c. Hypoglycemia with hypertension
    d. Weight gain associated with hyperglycemia

16. The nurse is teaching dietary planning to Mrs. Justice, 46 years old and newly diagnosed with diabetes. The nurse emphasizes the diet of a person with diabetes is very important. She stresses that 60% of the calories should come from:
    a. Proteins
    b. Refined sugars
    c. Unsaturated fats
    d. Complex carbohydrates

17. A bottle of insulin is labeled U-100. The nurse recognizes this as:
    a. 100 mg/unit
    b. 100 units/dose
    c. 100 units/bottle
    d. 100 units/ml

18. Mrs. Justice has been prescribed insulin. The nurse teaches that this insulin is rapid-acting with peak action between 2 and 4 hours. Mrs. Justice has been prescribed the following insulin:
    a. Lente
    b. Regular
    c. Semilente
    d. Ultralente

19. After insulin is injected, it takes some time for it to take effect; the period of time at which it has the strongest effect is the:
    a. Peak
    b. Limit
    c. Onset
    d. Duration

20. The most common signs of hypoglycemia are:
    a. Perspiration, faintness, weakness
    b. Hypotension, craving of sweet foods
    c. Hypertension, flushed effect, headaches
    d. Bradycardia, sudden emotional outbursts

21. The condition that results from a lack, or deficiency, of insulin is called:
    a. Insipidus
    b. Ketoacidosis
    c. Hypoglycemia
    d. Hyperglycemia

22. When a patient is prescribed a long-lasting insulin, he or she is given:
    a. NPH
    b. Lente
    c. Regular
    d. Ultralente

23. Mrs. Johnson is prescribed regular insulin along with an immediate-acting insulin. The other insulin is:
    a. NPH
    b. Regular
    c. Semilente
    d. Ultralente

24. A common complication of diabetes mellitus is:
    a. Hypotension
    b. Lactic acidosis
    c. Poor circulation
    d. Insulin reactions

25. Diabetes is the leading cause of blindness in the United States. This condition is called:
    a. Retina detachment
    b. Diabetic neuropathy
    c. Diabetic retinopathy
    d. Diabetic nephropathy

26. Mrs. Sims, 43 years old, was diagnosed several years ago with acromegaly and has lately complained of dyspnea. The nurse assesses tachycardia and hypotension. These signs and symptoms indicate:
    a. Idiopathic hyperplasia
    b. Respiratory failure
    c. Congestive heart failure
    d. Chronic fatigue syndrome

27. The nurse would make the following assessment in a patient with diabetic ketoacidosis:
    a. Fruity breath
    b. Frothy breath
    c. Sudden pallor
    d. Cheyne-Stokes breathing

28. Mrs. Dempsey, 68 years old, was diagnosed 8 months ago with pancreatic cancer. She has been hospitalized following an episode of weakness, anorexia, nausea, and headaches. She was diagnosed with the syndrome of inappropriate antidiuretic hormone (SIADH). The following nursing intervention is indicated:
    a. Force fluids
    b. Hypotonic IV infusion
    c. Diet emphasizing salty foods
    d. Neurological assessment every 3 to 4 hours

29. Mr. Glandon, 46 years old, has been prescribed regular insulin (Velosulin), 10 units/day. The most important time for him to observe for a hypoglycemic reaction is in:
    a. 1 to 3 hours
    b. 2 to 4 hours
    c. 3 to 6 hours
    d. 4 to 8 hours

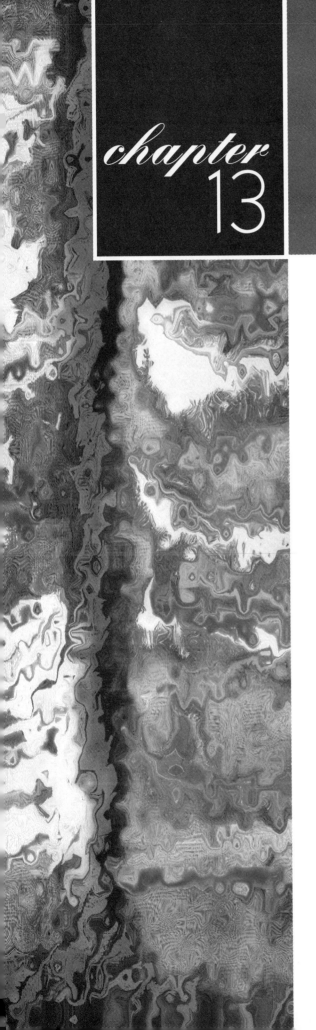

chapter 13

Care of the Patient with a Reproductive Disorder

CHAPTER SUMMARY

Chapter 13 describes the functions of the male and female reproductive systems in detail. Menstruation and the hormones involved in the menstrual cycle are described, as well as the nursing interventions required when a patient presents with menstrual disturbances. All other major reproductive disorders, including pelvic inflammatory disease (PID), endometriosis, cancer, hysterectomy, prostatitis, and sexually transmitted diseases, are detailed, with a focus on nursing diagnoses and interventions. There is a detailed focus on assessment of reproductive disorders and nursing interventions. Surgical interventions are also detailed.

LEARNING OBJECTIVES

After reading the chapter in the textbook and working through the chapter in this study guide, the student should be able to do the following:

Anatomy and Physiology

- List and describe the functions of the organs of the male and female reproductive tracts.
- Discuss menstruation and the hormones necessary for a complete cycle.

Medical-Surgical

- Define the key terms found in the matching exercises.
- Discuss the impact of illness on the patient's sexuality.
- List nursing interventions for patients with menstrual disturbances.
- Discuss nursing interventions for the patient undergoing diagnostic studies related to the reproductive system.
- Discuss the importance of the Papanicolaou smear test in early detection of cancer.
- Discuss four important points to be addressed in discharge planning for the patient with PID.
- List four nursing diagnoses pertinent to the patient with endometriosis.
- Identify the clinical manifestations seen with a vaginal fistula.
- Discuss the four major areas of postoperative concerns in the nursing interventions for a patient undergoing a hysterectomy.
- Identify four nursing diagnoses pertinent to ovarian cancer.
- Describe six important points to emphasize in the teaching of breast self-examination.
- Compare five surgical approaches for cancer of the breast.
- Discuss nursing interventions for the patient after a mastectomy.
- List several discharge planning instructions for the mastectomy patient.
- Describe nursing interventions for the patient with prostatitis.
- Distinguish between hydrocele and varicocele.
- Discuss the importance of monthly testicular self-examination beginning at 15 years of age.
- Discuss patient education related to prevention of sexually transmitted diseases.

KEY TERMS AND DEFINITIONS

_____ 1. Amenorrhea
_____ 2. Candidiasis
_____ 3. Carcinoma in situ
_____ 4. Chancre
_____ 5. *Chlamydia trachomatis*
_____ 6. Colporrhaphy
_____ 7. Colposcopy
_____ 8. Culdoscopy
_____ 9. Curettage
_____ 10. Dysmenorrhea
_____ 11. Endometriosis
_____ 12. Epididymitis
_____ 13. Fistula
_____ 14. Menorrhagia
_____ 15. Metrorrhagia
_____ 16. Trichomoniasis

a. An abnormal opening between two organs
b. Excessive menstrual flow
c. A direct visualization of the cervix and vagina
d. A mild fungal infection that appears in men and women; usually caused by *Candida albicans* or *Candida tropicalis*
e. A visualization of the uterus and adnexa (uterine appendages, ovaries, fallopian tubes, small intestine)
f. A condition in which endometrial tissue appears outside the uterus
g. A gram-negative, intracellular bacterium that causes several commonly sexually transmitted diseases
h. Surgical repair of the vaginal wall
i. Painful menstruation
j. Absence of menstrual flow
k. Scraping of material from the wall of a cavity or other surface (performed to remove tumors or other abnormal tissue for microscopic study)
l. A sexually transmitted disease caused by the protozoan *Trichomonas vaginalis*
m. The initial lesion of syphilis
n. An infection of the cordlike excretory duct of the testicles
o. Excessive spotting between menstrual cycles
p. A preinvasive, asymptomatic carcinoma that can only be diagnosed by microscopic examination of the cervical cells

REINFORCING KEY POINTS

1. Explain the function of the testes.

2. Explain what the hormone testosterone does.

3. Identify the anatomy of the male and female reproductive systems in the figures below:

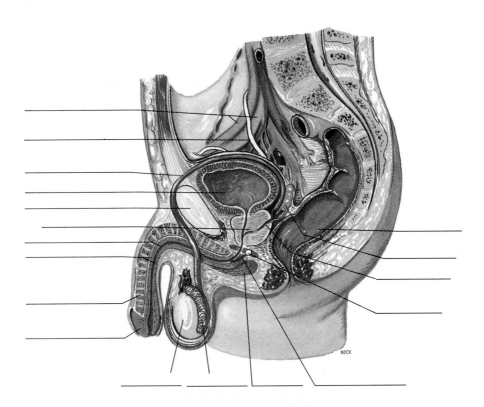

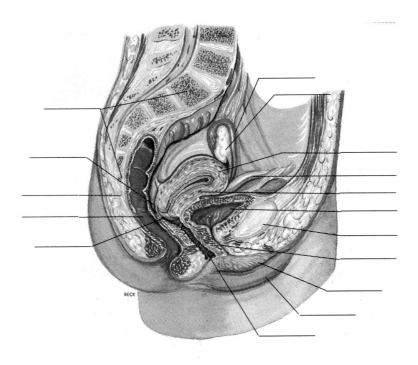

4. Describe the menstrual cycle, including ovulation and how hormones activate and regulate this process.

5. Describe the normal effects of aging on the reproductive system.

6. Define the following dysfunctions of the menstrual cycle:
   a. Amenorrhea

   b. Menorrhagia

   c. Metrorrhagia

   d. Dysmenorrhea

7. Explain what human chorionic gonadotropin (HCG) is and why it is the basis for all pregnancy tests.

8. Discuss nursing interventions appropriate for the patient undergoing diagnostic tests of the reproductive system.

9. Discuss the possible cause of premenstrual syndrome (PMS), its symptoms, and nursing interventions.

10. Outline the clinical manifestations of menopause and what the menopausal woman can do to deal with these symptoms.

11. Cite major causes for impotence, possible interventions, diagnostic tests, and medications.

12. Cite the cause and medical management for these infections of the female reproductive tract:
    a. Vaginitis

    b. Cervicitis

    c. *Trichomonas*

    d. Toxic shock syndrome

    e. Pelvic inflammatory disease (PID)

13. Explain how toxic shock syndrome can be prevented.

14. Explain what endometriosis is, including medical management.

15. List conditions that result because of relaxed pelvic muscles.

16. Discuss nursing interventions and patient teaching for the post-hysterectomy patient.

17. Discuss the factors that predispose some women to breast cancer.

18. Discuss the recommended nursing interventions related to the nursing diagnosis of body image disturbance.

19. Discuss the clinical manifestations and medical management in the following male reproductive disorders:
    a. Phimosis

b. Prostatitis

c. Hydrocele

d. Varicocele

e. Epididymitis

20. Describe the clinical manifestations and medical management of the following sexually transmitted diseases:
   a. Syphilis

   b. Gonorrhea

   c. Candidiasis

   d. Trichomoniasis

   e. Herpes genitalis

   f. Chlamydial infection

APPLICATION OF CLINICAL SKILLS

1. Prepare a patient teaching plan for a female on how to prevent sexually transmitted diseases.

2. Prepare a patient teaching plan describing the menstrual cycle and the hormones that activate the cycle.

3. Describe how sex and sexuality differ and the implications this difference holds for nursing.

4. Explain methods of contraception to a young couple who wants to delay parenthood.

5. Instruct a patient on how to do Kegel exercises.

6. Instruct a male patient on how to do a testicular examination for cancer.

EXERCISES IN FUNDAMENTAL CONCEPTS

1. The testes also produce _____, which is responsible for the development of male secondary sex characteristics.

2. Mature sperm, once deposited in the female reproductive system, live approximately _____.

3. During the menstrual cycle, an ovum matures and is released about _____ before the next menstrual flow. This, on average, occurs every _____.

4. _____ is often described as the sense of being female or male.

5. _____ usually describes the biological aspects of sexuality, such as genital sexual activity.

6. Gender identity is the _____.
   Gender role is the _____.

7. Painful menstruation is called _____, whereas excessive flow is called _____.

8. _____ are procedures in which samples of tissues are taken for evaluation to confirm or locate a lesion.

9. _____ of the cervix is indicated when eroded or infected tissue is to be removed or there is a need for confirmation of cervical cancer.

10. All pregnancy tests, regardless of the method, are based on detection of _____, which is secreted in the urine after fertilization of the ovum.

11. The _____ is the phase of the aging process of women and men who are making a transition from a reproductive phase to a nonreproductive phase of life. The female climacteric is called _____.

12. _____ is a condition in which endometrial tissue appears outside the uterus.

13. _____ is sexual intercourse accompanied by pain.

14. A _____ is defined as an abnormal opening between two organs and is named for the organs involved.

15. _____ is an opening between the urethra and vagina.

16. _____ is an opening between the bladder and vagina.

17. _____ is an opening between the rectum and vagina.

18. A hysterectomy involves the removal of the _____, including the _____. A total abdominal hysterectomy with bilateral salpingooophorectomy (TAH-BSO) is the removal of the _____, _____, and _____.

19. _____ is a preinvasive, asymptomatic carcinoma that can only be diagnosed by microscopic examination of cervical cells.

EXERCISES IN CRITICAL THINKING

Topics for Writing

1. Sketch a diagram showing the events that occur during the 28-day menstrual cycle, including the changes in body temperature.

2. Describe the effects of aging on the sexual response.

Topics for Discussion

1. Discuss factors that interfere with the practice of good health related to sex.

2. Discuss the implications of the male climacteric, including the nursing interventions that are appropriate when addressing this issue with the male patient.

3. Consider emotional support for the woman who is preparing for a hysterectomy.

4. Consider emotional support for the woman who has been diagnosed with breast cancer and has had a mastectomy.

STUDY QUESTIONS

1. The organ in the reproductive system that produces sperm is the:
   a. Penis
   b. Testes
   c. Vas deferens
   d. Ejaculatory ducts

2. The following is the male hormone:
   a. Estrogen
   b. Testosterone
   c. Progesterone
   d. Growth hormone

3. Mrs. Davis, 26 years old, has just confirmed her first pregnancy. The nurse explains that in the process of conception the union of the sperm and ovum occurs in the:
   a. Uterus
   b. Cervix
   c. Vagina
   d. Fallopian tubes

4. The chief advantage of mammography is:
   a. It has no side effects
   b. It is a painless procedure
   c. It detects malignant lesions early
   d. It is 100% accurate

5. After menopause there is a decrease in a hormone, and this can lead to hot flashes, vaginal atrophy, and osteoporosis. The hormone is:
   a. Estrogen
   b. Androgen
   c. Testosterone
   d. Progesterone

6. Osteoporosis is a disorder commonly seen in postmenopausal women. The dietary supplement recommended to retard and even reverse this condition is:
   a. Calcium
   b. Vitamin D
   c. Vitamin A
   d. Phosphorus

7. Mrs. Simmons, 22 years old, has been experiencing the pain associated with chronic pelvic inflammatory disease. This patient often seeks medical care for:
   a. Pain
   b. Infertility
   c. Hemorrhage
   d. Dyspareunia

8. Miss Butler, 16 years old, is at highest risk for toxic shock syndrome. On assessment, this determination was made because she:
   a. Experiences untreated chronic PID
   b. Has had multiple abortions
   c. Inserts tampons with her fingers
   d. Has multiple sexual contacts

9. Miss Reynolds, 17 years old, has just been diagnosed with toxic shock syndrome after being taken to the emergency room. The first significant sign of toxic shock syndrome that a patient will exhibit is:
   a. Foul vaginal odor
   b. Sudden high fever
   c. Sudden hypotension
   d. Vaginal hemorrhage

10. The bacterium associated with toxic shock syndrome is:
    a. *Escherichia coli*
    b. *Candida albicans*
    c. *Staphylococcus aureus*
    d. *Staphylococcus pyogenes*

11. Abdominal and low back pain that specifically increases in severity during menstruation is a sign of the following disorder:
    a. Endometriosis
    b. Ovarian tumor
    c. Uterine cancer
    d. Cervical polyp

12. The position to be avoided after a hysterectomy for the first 24 hours is:
    a. Prone
    b. Fowler's
    c. Completely flat
    d. Supine with knees up

13. The following patient action will prevent complications of hysterectomy, such as constipation and thrombosis:
    a. Active range of motion (ROM)
    b. Early voiding
    c. Early ambulation
    d. Optimistic attitude

14. An early sign of breast cancer is:
    a. Dimpling of the skin
    b. Small, palpable mass
    c. Discharge from nipple
    d. Distortion of the nipple

15. The woman at highest risk for breast cancer has:
    a. A mother with breast cancer
    b. Menarche after 13 years old
    c. Menopause before 40 years old
    d. Given birth before the age of 20

16. The prostate gland is important clinically because it has an affinity for inflammation, hyperplasia, and malignancy. Because of its anatomical position, prostatic problems often present as:
    a. Low back pain
    b. Rectal bleeding
    c. Penile erections
    d. Urinary tract symptoms

17. Mrs. Baxter is complaining of pelvic discomfort and describes it as "something coming down." She has also experienced stress incontinence. She is experiencing:
    a. Vaginal fistula
    b. Uterine prolapse
    c. Bladder irritation
    d. Rectovaginal fistula

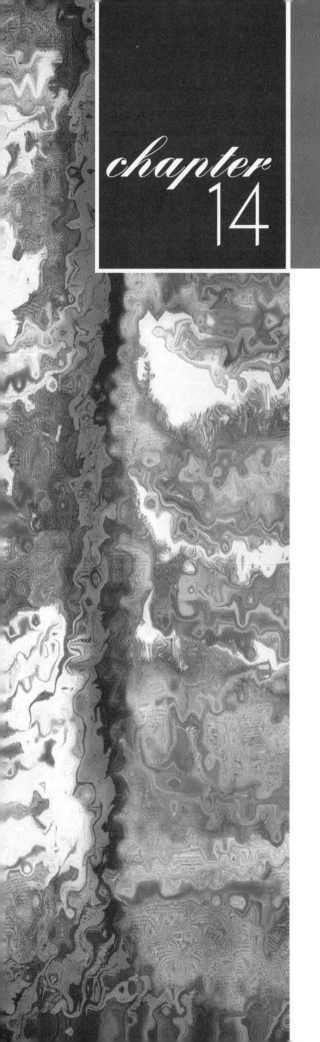

chapter 14

Care of the Patient with an Eye and Ear Disorder

CHAPTER SUMMARY

Chapter 14 describes the anatomy of the eye and ear, in addition to the function of each part. The techniques for assessing the eye and ear are detailed, as well as the purposes and procedures for diagnostic tests of the sensory organs. Signs and symptoms of disorders, such as cataracts, inflammation, and retinal detachment, as well as nursing interventions, are included.

LEARNING OBJECTIVES

After reading the chapter in the textbook and working through the chapter in this study guide, the student should be able to do the following:

Anatomy and Physiology

- List the major sense organs, and discuss their anatomical position.
- List the parts of the eye, and define the function of each part.
- List the three divisions of the ear, and discuss the function of each.

Medical-Surgical

- Define the key terms found in the matching exercises.
- Describe two changes in the sensory system that occur as a result of the normal aging process.
- Describe the techniques used in assessment of the eye and ear.
- Identify the purposes and procedures for diagnostic tests of the eye and ear.
- Describe major eye inflammations and appropriate nursing interventions.
- Compare the nature of cataracts, glaucoma, and retinal detachment and appropriate nursing interventions for each.
- Identify the nursing interventions associated with medical-surgical treatment of the eye and ear.
- Differentiate between conductive and sensorineural hearing loss.
- List communication tips for hearing- and sight-impaired persons.
- Give patient instructions regarding care of the eye and ear in accordance with written protocol.
- Describe appropriate nursing interventions for the patient having eye and ear surgery.
- Identify communication resources for persons with visual or hearing impairment or both.
- Describe home health considerations for persons with eye or ear disorders, surgery, or visual and hearing impairments.

KEY TERMS AND DEFINITIONS

_____ 1. Astigmatism
_____ 2. Cataract
_____ 3. Conjunctivitis
_____ 4. Cryosurgery
_____ 5. Diabetic retinopathy
_____ 6. Enucleation
_____ 7. Glaucoma
_____ 8. Keratoplasty
_____ 9. Labyrinthitis
_____ 10. Mastoiditis
_____ 11. Mydriatic
_____ 12. Myopia
_____ 13. Myringotomy
_____ 14. Strabismus
_____ 15. Tinnitus
_____ 16. Tympanoplasty

a. Defect in the curvature of the eyeball surface
b. Surgery to excise an opaque portion of the cornea
c. Surgical incision of the eardrum
d. Tingling or ringing in one or both ears
e. A disorder of retinal blood vessels characterized by capillary microaneurysm, hemorrhage, and formation of new vessels; may appear 10 years after onset of diabetes mellitus
f. Condition of nearsightedness; inability to see objects at a distance
g. Surgical procedure performed on the eardrum to restore or improve hearing in patients with conductive deafness
h. Inflammation of the conjunctiva
i. Elevated pressure within the eye caused by obstruction of the outflow of aqueous humor
j. Cross-eye
k. Infection of one of the mastoid bones
l. Inflammation of the inner ear canal resulting in vertigo
m. Opacity or clouding of the lens
n. Surgical removal of the eyeball
o. Causing dilation of the pupil of the eye
p. Use of subfreezing temperature to destroy tissue

REINFORCING KEY POINTS

1. Explain how eye blinking protects the eye.

2. Define "lazy eye."

3. Describe the structure of the eyeball, including the:
   a. Iris

   b. Pupil

   c. Sclera

   d. Cornea

e. Choroid

f. Canal of Schlemm

4. Explain what causes color blindness.

5. Explain the meaning of accommodation.

6. Identify the anatomy of the external, middle, and
    internal ear in the figure below:

7. Define the following terms:
    a. Myopia

    b. Hyperopia

    c. Strabismus

    d. Presbyopia

    e. Astigmatism

    f. Exophthalmos

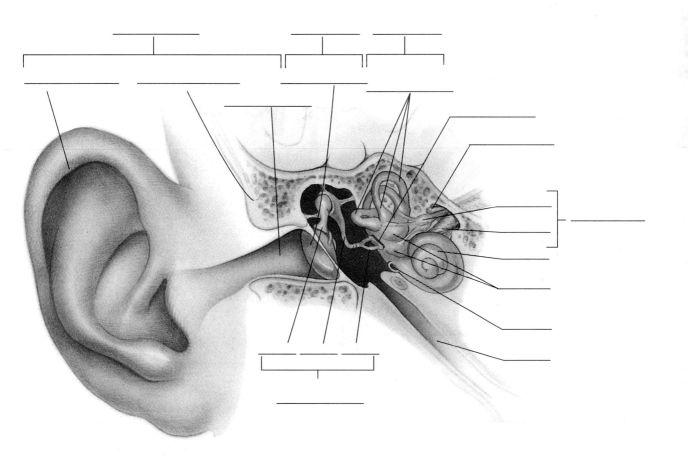

8. Describe the etiology and medical management for conjunctivitis, or pinkeye.

9. Describe an assessment of a cataract.

10. Describe the nursing care of the patient with an eye disorder.

11. Describe the symptoms of a retinal detachment.

12. Discuss the assessment and medical management of glaucoma.

13. Describe the first-aid measures for the following eye injuries:
   a. Dirt, insects

   b. Contact injury

   c. Penetrating objects

   d. Burns: chemical, flame

14. Discuss the six types of hearing loss.

15. Discuss how communication for a person with impaired hearing can be facilitated.

16. Describe the assessment and medical management for the patient with otitis media.

17. Describe the postoperative care of a patient with Meniere's disease.

APPLICATION OF CLINICAL SKILLS

1. Give instructions on how to communicate with a blind person.

2. Explain techniques that facilitate communication with the hearing impaired.

3. Write a teaching plan for a patient with glaucoma, including medications and how to prevent complications.

4. Describe how to avoid eye strain.

5. Describe the teaching appropriate for a patient with an ear infection.

6. Teach the patient what precautions should be taken after eye surgery.

7. Instruct a patient on how to care for a hearing aid.

EXERCISES IN FUNDAMENTAL CONCEPTS

1. The accessory structures of the eye—the eyebrows, eyelashes, eyelids, and lacrimal apparatus—function mainly as _____.

2. The _____ is a thin mucous membrane that lines the inner aspect of the eyelids and the anterior surface of the eyeball to the edge of the cornea.

3. The outermost layer of the eyeball is the fibrous tunic, composed of thick, white, opaque, connective tissue called the _____, or white of the eye.

4. Intraocular pressure is the _____ within the _____.

5. A circular opening in the iris of the eye, located slightly to the nasal side of the center of the iris, is the _____.

6. The _____ is a 10-layered, delicate, nervous tissue membrane of the eye that receives images of external objects and transmits impulses through the optic nerve to the brain.

7. _____ is the bending of light rays as they pass through the colorless structures of the eye, allowing light from the environment to focus on the retina.

8. _____ is the adjustment of the eye for various distances; thus it is able to focus the image of an object on the retina by changing the curvature of the lens.

9. _____ is the movement of both eyes medially to allow light rays from an object to hit the same point on both retinas.

10. The _____ is lined with mucous membrane that joins the nasopharynx and the middle ear cavity. It is also called the auditory canal.

11. _____ are any sensory nerve endings, such as those located in muscles, tendons, and joints, that respond to stimuli originating from within the body regarding movement and spatial position; they work in conjunction with the semicircular canals and vestibule of the inner ear to maintain proper coordination.

12. _____ is an abnormal condition characterized by a marked protrusion of the eyeballs.

EXERCISES IN CRITICAL THINKING

Topics for Writing

1. Explain what accommodation means and its implications in doing a physical assessment.

2. List the initial nursing considerations for a patient with an eye disorder.

Topics for Discussion

1. Discuss the multiple changes that occur to the eyes during the aging process.

2. Discuss the guidelines for communicating with a blind patient.

3. Discuss the emotional support that the nurse can provide in facilitating communication with the hearing-impaired patient.

STUDY QUESTIONS

1. The eye must make adjustments when seeing objects at different distances. This is called:
   a. Myopia
   b. Cataract
   c. Refraction
   d. Accommodation

2. Mr. Johnson, 68 years old, is being tested for distance vision using the Snellen chart. The nurse asks Mr. Johnson to stand at a distance of:
   a. 12 inches
   b. 20 inches
   c. 20 feet
   d. 30 feet

3. Mr. Johnson is standing at the proper distance to use the Snellen chart. The nurse then asks him to:
   a. Use only one eye at a time
   b. Read the chart from right to left
   c. Cover one eye while testing the other
   d. Use both eyes when reading the chart

4. An alteration in visual acuity in which light rays focus in front of the retina is called:
   a. Myopia
   b. Hyperopia
   c. Refraction
   d. Presbyopia

5. The eye medication that causes the pupil to dilate is:
   a. Miotic
   b. Myopic
   c. Osmotic
   d. Mydriatic

6. Mrs. Atkins, 73 years old, is blind. The best way for the nurse to assist her walking is to:
   a. Take the blind person's left arm
   b. Take the blind person's right arm
   c. Lead the blind person with both hands
   d. Precede the blind person by about 1 foot and have the person's hand on the nurse's elbow

7. Mr. Johnson, 72 years old, is complaining of difficulty seeing when the lens of the eye becomes cloudy and opaque. The condition is called:
   a. Normal
   b. Cataract
   c. Glaucoma
   d. Presbyopia

8. Mrs. Beebe, 68 years old, has just been diagnosed with glaucoma. She asks, "What causes it, isn't it rare?" The nurse explains that the cause of glaucoma is:
   a. Infection of the lens
   b. Clouding of the lens
   c. Separation of the retina
   d. Obstruction of aqueous humor drainage

9. In instructing Mrs. Beebe regarding self-care, the nurse emphasizes that she will:
   a. Never use miotic eye drops
   b. Never use reading eyeglasses
   c. Read for only 20 minutes at a time
   d. Continue to see her doctor for the rest of her life

10. The patient complains of a halo around lights; the nurse suspects that this patient is experiencing:
    a. Cataracts
    b. Glaucoma
    c. Presbyopia
    d. Retinal detachment

11. Medications that constrict the pupil are:
    a. Miotic
    b. Myopic
    c. Inhibitors
    d. Mydriatic

12. In caring for the patient with a foreign object in the cornea, the priority nursing intervention is to:
    a. Gently wipe out the foreign body
    b. Pull out the object immediately
    c. Cover loosely and call the physician
    d. Immediately irrigate with tap water

13. The nurse instructs the patient who uses ophthalmic solutions to watch for discoloration in the medication. The patient is instructed to discard the bottle of medication if:
    a. It has been in the refrigerator
    b. It has been sealed for 2 months
    c. It has been opened for 6 months
    d. All particles have been dissolved

14. The most common problem of the external ear is external otitis. This occurs:
    a. Mostly in adults
    b. Mostly in the North
    c. Mostly in the winter
    d. Mostly in the summer

15. A major symptom of an inner ear disorder is:
    a. Echoes
    b. Dizziness
    c. Severe pain
    d. Hearing loss

16. Inner ear problems often cause dizziness, which is a common health complaint. The medical term for dizziness is:
    a. Acuity
    b. Vertigo
    c. Tinnitus
    d. Mydriasis

17. The priority nursing interventions in caring for a patient who is dizzy concern:
    a. Pain
    b. Safety
    c. Nausea
    d. Vomiting

18. After ear surgery, the most common symptom the nurse must be alert for is:
    a. Bleeding
    b. Insomnia
    c. Dizziness
    d. Discomfort

19. Postoperative care for the patient who has just undergone a stapedectomy includes correct positioning. The nurse places this patient:
    a. Prone with face up
    b. Supine with face to side
    c. On side with operative ear up
    d. On side with operative ear down

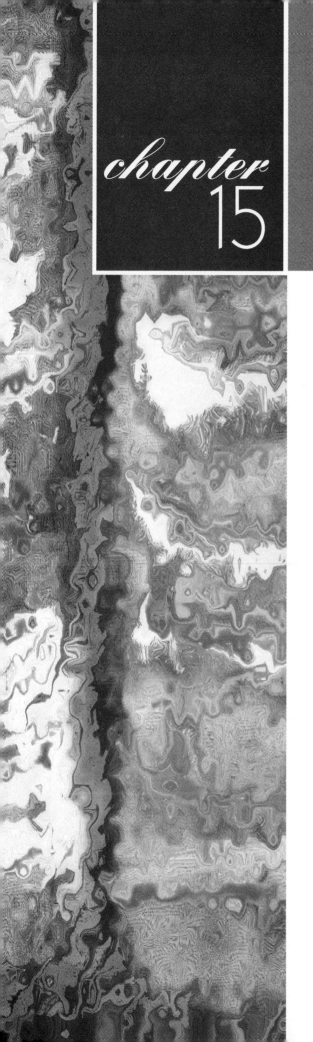

chapter 15

Care of the Patient with a Neurological Disorder

CHAPTER SUMMARY

Chapter 15 describes in extensive detail the nervous system and its physiology. The anatomy of the neuron, the brain, and the cranial nerves is described. Conditions of the neurological system, including the physiological changes of aging and increased intracranial pressure, are covered, with emphasis on nursing interventions. The importance of the neurological assessment and what that assessment entails are covered, along with the measures that are recommended in preventing neurological problems and complications.

LEARNING OBJECTIVES

After reading the chapter in the textbook and working through the chapter in this study guide, the student should be able to do the following:

Anatomy and Physiology
- Define the key terms found in the matching exercises.
- Name the two structural divisions of the nervous system, and give the function of each.
- List the parts of the neuron, and describe the function of each part.
- List the main parts and coverings of the brain.
- Discuss the parts of the peripheral nervous system and how the system works with the central nervous system.
- Name the 12 cranial nerves, and list the areas they serve.

Medical-Surgical

- Define the key terms found in the matching exercises.
- List physiological changes that occur in the nervous system with aging.
- Discuss the Glasgow Coma Scale.
- Explain three parts of the neurological assessment.
- Explain the importance of prevention in problems of the nervous system, and give at least one example of prevention.
- List five signs and symptoms of increased intracranial pressure and why they occur as well as nursing interventions that decrease intracranial pressure.
- Give examples of two degenerative neurological diseases and two diseases related to infection of the nervous system, and explain the pathophysiology involved.
- State two complications of brain surgery and the signs and symptoms seen with each complication.
- Explain the mechanism of injury to the brain that occurs with cerebrovascular accident and traumatic brain injury.
- Discuss nursing interventions to assist in the rehabilitation of the patient with a cerebrovascular accident.
- Discuss patient teaching and home care planning for the patient with multiple sclerosis or Parkinson's disease.
- Discuss the pathophysiology of Guillain-Barré syndrome, trigeminal neuralgia, and Bell's palsy.
- Contrast and compare amyotrophic lateral sclerosis and Huntington's disease.

KEY TERMS AND DEFINITIONS

_____	1. Aneurysm
_____	2. Aphasia
_____	3. Apraxia
_____	4. Dysarthria
_____	5. Dysphagia
_____	6. Hemianopia
_____	7. Hemiplegia
_____	8. Hyperreflexia
_____	9. Nystagmus
_____	10. Postictal period
_____	11. Proprioception
_____	12. Unilateral neglect

a. A neurological condition characterized by increased reflex actions

b. An impairment in the ability to perform purposeful acts, often seen in Alzheimer's disease

c. The rest period following an epileptic seizure during which the patient usually feels groggy and confused and may experience amnesia for the event

d. A condition by which an individual is perceptually unaware of and inattentive to one side of the body

e. Difficult, poorly articulated speech that usually results from interference in the control of the muscles of speech

f. Paralysis on one side of the body

g. An abnormal neurological condition in which the language function is defective or absent because of an injury to certain areas of the cerebral cortex

h. A condition characterized by defective vision or blindness in one half of the visual field

i. The sensation pertaining to stimuli originating from within the body regarding spatial position and muscular activity or to the sensory receptors that they activate; this sensation gives one the ability to know the position of the body without looking at it and the ability to "know" objects by the sense of touch

j. Severe swallowing difficulty that commonly results from obstructive or motor disorders of the esophagus and is commonly associated with neurological problems

k. Involuntary, rhythmic movement of the eyes; oscillations may be horizontal, vertical, rotary, or mixed

l. A localized dilation of the wall of a blood vessel usually caused by atherosclerosis and hypertension or, less frequently, by trauma, infection, or a congenital weakness in the vessel wall

REINFORCING KEY POINTS

1. Describe the two main structural divisions of the nervous system: the central nervous system and the peripheral nervous system.

2. Differentiate between sensory neurons (nerve cells) and motor neurons.

3. Describe the functioning of the autonomic nervous system.

4. Describe the function of neurons.

5. Describe the functions of the three structures of the neuron: the cell body, dendrites, and axons.

6. Explain what happens at the synapse.

7. Note the functions of the 12 pairs of cranial nerves. Discuss the role of the following cranial nerves:
   a. Trigeminal

   b. Glossopharyngeal

   c. Vagus

   d. Spinal accessory

8. Describe the special functions that the frontal lobe performs.

9. Discuss the action of afferent neurons and efferent neurons.

10. Discuss the transmission of nerve impulses.

11. Briefly discuss the functions of these parts of the brain:
    a. Pons

    b. Cerebrum

    c. Brain stem

    d. Cerebellum

    e. Diencephalon

    f. Hypothalamus

    g. Medulla oblongata

12. Describe how the spinal cord controls reflexes in the body.

13. Discuss how the autonomic nervous system is divided into two parts, and describe the function of each.

14. Differentiate the three kinds of aphasia—sensory, motor, and global. Give an example of each.

15. Explain the purpose of a lumbar puncture.

16. Discuss the common complication that occurs after a lumbar puncture and the nursing interventions that are recommended.

17. Describe the purpose and preparation for the following diagnostic tests:
    a. Angiogram

    b. Myelogram

    c. Electromyogram

    d. Electroencephalogram

18. Outline the prodromal signs and symptoms of a migraine headache.

19. Name the foods that are associated with the occurrence of headaches.

20. Discuss the options available when a patient is suffering intractable pain.

21. Discuss the early signs of increased intracranial pressure.

22. Describe the assessment and significance of a "blown pupil."

23. Differentiate the characteristics of the following seizures:
    a. Akinetic

    b. Myoclonic

    c. Psychomotor

    d. Jacksonian (focal)

24. Discuss the signs and symptoms of multiple sclerosis.

25. Discuss who is at greatest risk to be diagnosed with multiple sclerosis and the nursing interventions that can be implemented.

26. Describe the clinical manifestations of Parkinson's disease.

27. Describe the signs and symptoms of Alzheimer's disease and nursing interventions for this disease.

28. Discuss the factors that increase the risk of stroke.

29. Describe the etiology and medical management of meningitis.

30. Describe the neurological manifestations of acquired immunodeficiency syndrome (AIDS).

APPLICATION OF CLINICAL SKILLS

1. In assessing a patient with neurological problems the nurse should gather specific subjective data. Outline the questions that should be asked.

2. Discuss the assessment data that are documented for the following levels of consciousness:
   a. Alert
   b. Stupor
   c. Comatose
   d. Confusion
   e. Semicomatose

3. Discuss nursing interventions required for the person who suffers headaches.

4. Instruct a patient on how a transcutaneous electrical nerve stimulation (TENS) unit works.

5. List the 10 conservative nursing interventions the nurse can take to reduce venous volume in the patient with increased intracranial pressure.

6. Assess the patient whose eyes open to speech, who is confused, and who localizes pain.

7. Demonstrate the position for the patient who is scheduled for a lumbar puncture.

8. Demonstrate decorticate posturing and decerebrate posturing.

EXERCISES IN FUNDAMENTAL CONCEPTS

1. The first division, the _____, is composed of the _____ and the _____.

2. The second component is the _____, which lies outside the central nervous system (CNS).

3. The autonomic system is sometimes called the _____ because its action takes place without conscious control.

4. There are _____ of spinal nerves and _____ of cranial nerves.

5. The primary function of the _____ is to maintain internal homeostasis; for example, it strives to maintain a normal heartbeat, a constant body temperature, and a normal respiratory pattern.

6. The autonomic system has two divisions: the _____ and the _____.

7. A decreasing level of consciousness is the earliest sign of _____.

8. The _____ consists of testing of three parts of the neurological assessment: eye opening, best motor response, and best verbal response.

9. A loss of function is called _____; a lesser degree of movement deficit is called _____.

10. A pupil that is fixed and dilated is sometimes called a _____ and is an ominous sign that must be reported to the physician immediately.

11. A widened pulse pressure, increased systolic blood pressure, and bradycardia are together called _____.

12. _____ is paralysis of one side of the body.

13. _____ is a total or partial loss of the ability to recognize familiar objects or persons through sensory stimuli as a result of organic brain damage.

14. _____ is a sensation, as of light or warmth, that may precede an attack of migraine or an epileptic seizure.

15. _____ is an involuntary, rhythmic movement of the eye; the oscillation may be horizontal, vertical, rotary, or mixed.

16. _____ is an abnormal condition characterized by slowness of voluntary movements and speech and is present with rigidity and loss of postural reflexes.

17. _____ is impairment in the ability to perform purposeful acts and interferes with the ability to carry out daily functions.

18. When a patient fails to recognize that he or she has a paralyzed side, it is called

_____ .

19. Quadriplegics are patients who sustain injuries to _____ of the cervical segments of the spinal cord. Paraplegics are those whose lesions are confined to the _____, _____, or _____ segments of the spinal cord.

20. _____ is a neurological condition characterized by increased reflex actions.

21. _____ occurs as a result of abnormal cardiovascular response to stimulation of the sympathetic division of the autonomic nervous system as a result of stimulation of the bladder, large intestine, or other visceral organs.

EXERCISES IN CRITICAL THINKING

Topics for Writing

1. List the major functions of the sympathetic nervous system and the parasympathetic nervous system.

2. Give some ideas on how neurological problems can be prevented, especially related to accidents.

3. List the components of a neurological history, and briefly remark as to why each component is important to explore.

Topics for Discussion

1. Using the information that you gain from listing the major functions of the sympathetic and parasympathetic nervous systems, discuss how each system balances the other and what this means to day-to-day body functioning.

2. Explore your ideas on how enkephalins and endorphins work as the body's pain relievers and affect other areas of our lives, such as memory and learning and sexual activity.

3. Differentiate among migraine, cluster, and tension headaches, including triggering factors.

4. Discuss why patient teaching is so important when caring for a neurological patient, including examples of lifestyle changes.

5. Discuss the possible implications regarding sexual function in the male and/or female who experiences a spinal cord injury.

STUDY QUESTIONS

1. Sue Brown, a nursing student, is caring for a patient with a head injury. What nursing intervention is contraindicated in the presence of an acute head injury?
   a. Turning from side to side
   b. Range-of-motion exercises
   c. Suctioning through the nose
   d. Elevating head of bed 30 degrees

2. Mrs. Smith, 85 years old, is admitted to a nursing home. The nurse knows that she or he can expect to see some normal aging changes. Which of the following is not a normal aging change of the neurological system?
   a. Altered sleep/wakefulness ratio
   b. Decrease in weight of the brain
   c. Senile changes in mental ability
   d. Reduction in cerebral blood flow

3. Timothy Jones is an 11-year-old adolescent admitted with a head injury sustained while driving a three-wheeler on his ranch. He is demonstrating a decreased level of consciousness. The physician orders a Glasgow Coma Scale every 3 hours. The Glasgow Coma Scale is a simple instrument to systematically assess level of consciousness. It is based on the patient's response in three major areas:
   a. Eye, pain, and verbal
   b. Eye, motor, and verbal
   c. Verbal, pain, and reflexes
   d. Verbal, sensation, and motor

4. Jack Thomas is a 26-year-old male who suffered a spinal cord injury that has left him a quadriplegic. Mr. Thomas at times has problems with autonomic dysreflexia. Which of the following is not indicative of autonomic dysreflexia?
   a. Diaphoresis
   b. Bradycardia
   c. Hypotension
   d. Severe headache

5. Mr. Lamberty has a history of grand mal seizures and experiences a warning feeling before a seizure. This is called a (an):
   a. Aura
   b. Tonicity
   c. Postictal
   d. Convulsion

6. Robert Jones has advanced Parkinson's disease. Which of the following is often a complication seen in patients with Parkinson's disease?
   a. Total paralysis
   b. Sjogren's syndrome
   c. Increasing spasticity
   d. Aspiration pneumonia

7. Ms. Josea was admitted for observation after being thrown out of her vehicle and sustaining a head injury. She has been alert and oriented and after several days becomes less responsive. What should be suspected?
   a. Skull fracture
   b. Ruptured aneurysm
   c. Epidural hematoma
   d. Subdural hematoma

8. Mrs. Evans is a 46-year-old patient with a 13-year history of progressively deteriorating multiple sclerosis. Which nursing intervention would not be appropriate for Mrs. Evans?
   a. Giving a hot bath to ensure cleanliness
   b. Taking the patient to the bathroom frequently
   c. Encouraging fluids to prevent urinary infection
   d. Using a suppository to help evacuate the bowel

9. Mrs. Willard is a 32-year-old patient with a spinal cord injury at C6. She often has signs and symptoms resulting from autonomic dysreflexia. The nurse can rule out which of the following as a cause of her autonomic dysreflexia:
   a. Kinked catheter
   b. Bowel impaction
   c. Urinary infection
   d. Postural hypotension

10. What is the first nursing intervention that is necessary in caring for the patient who has autonomic dysreflexia?
   a. Sit the patient upright
   b. Check for bowel impaction
   c. Give medication as ordered
   d. Place the patient in a supine position

11. The transmitter cells are called:
   a. Glials
   b. Axons
   c. Neurons
   d. Neuroglias

12. The part of the cell that branches out to receive impulses is the:
   a. Axon
   b. Neuron
   c. Dendrite
   d. Transmitter

13. The neurotransmitter that induces sleep and also plays a role in controlling moods is (are):
   a. Serotonin
   b. Endorphins
   c. Acetylcholine
   d. Norepinephrine

14. The lobe of the cerebrum that controls the ability to speak and to write is the:
   a. Parietal
   b. Frontal
   c. Occipital
   d. Temporal

15. The part of the brain that contains the respiratory center and regulates heartbeat is the:
   a. Midbrain
   b. Cerebellum
   c. Hypothalamus
   d. Medulla oblongata

16. The cranial nerve that controls the movements of the tongue is the:
    a. Olfactory
    b. Oculomotor
    c. Hypoglossal
    d. Glossopharyngeal

17. The cranial nerve that controls hearing and a sense of balance is the:
    a. Vagus
    b. Acoustic
    c. Trochlear
    d. Abducens

18. The nervous system that takes over to prepare the body for "fight or flight" during periods of stress is the:
    a. Peripheral nervous system
    b. Autonomic nervous system
    c. Sympathetic nervous system
    d. Parasympathetic nervous system

19. The following indicates parasympathetic control:
    a. Dilation of pupils
    b. Increased peristalsis
    c. Accelerated heartbeat
    d. Constriction of blood vessels

20. In assessing level of consciousness, the nurse finds the patient responding to verbal commands with moaning and groaning. The level of consciousness is:
    a. Stupor
    b. Comatose
    c. Confusion
    d. Semicomatose

21. Nursing interventions after a myelogram depend on:
    a. The kind of dye injected
    b. The physician's postoperative orders
    c. The results of the lumbar puncture (LP)
    d. How the patient tolerated the procedure

22. In assessing the first signs and symptoms of intracranial pressure, the subjective sign or symptom that would alert the nurse is:
    a. Seizures
    b. Diplopia
    c. Restlessness
    d. Hypertension

23. The headache that is caused by increased intracranial pressure will most often occur:
    a. Late at night
    b. Late in evening
    c. Early in morning
    d. Spontaneously at midday

24. The nursing assessment is as follows: fixed posture with arms, legs, and trunk extended and with flexion of the palms and plantar joints. The patient's posturing is:
    a. Ataxia
    b. Seizuring
    c. Decorticate
    d. Decerebrate

25. The focus of nursing care for the person who is having a seizure is to:
    a. Protect from injury
    b. Prevent another seizure
    c. Start oxygen immediately
    d. Prepare to administer drugs

26. The focus of nursing care for the patient with Alzheimer's disease is to:
    a. Provide safety
    b. Prevent disorientation
    c. Administer medications
    d. Provide emotional support

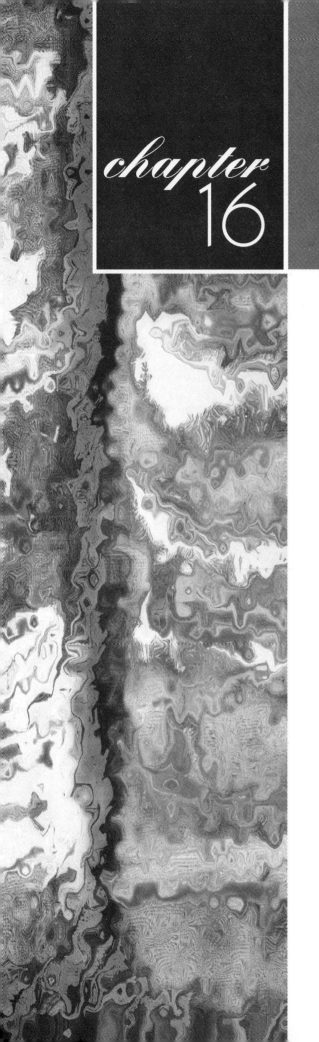

chapter 16

Care of Patient with HIV Disease

CHAPTER SUMMARY

Chapter 16 discusses the clinical manifestations of human immunodeficiency virus (HIV) disease. The chapter focuses on how HIV disease is transmitted, what the causative agent is, and how HIV disease can be prevented, especially among high-risk groups. Diagnostic tests, treatment modalities, and supportive care are discussed. A detailed nursing care plan is also presented.

LEARNING OBJECTIVES

After reading the chapter in the textbook and working through the chapter in this study guide, the student should be able to do the following:

- Define key terms found in the matching exercises.
- Describe the agent that causes HIV disease.
- Relate the January 1993 Centers for Disease Control and Prevention (CDC) definition of acquired immunodeficiency syndrome (AIDS).
- Describe the progression of HIV infection.
- Discuss how HIV is transmitted and how it is not transmitted.
- Discuss the pathophysiology of HIV disease.
- Discuss the laboratory and diagnostic tests related to HIV disease.
- Describe patients who are at risk for HIV infection.

- Discuss the use of effective prevention messages in counseling patients.
- Discuss the issues related to HIV antibody testing.
- Define the nurse's role in prevention of HIV infection.
- Discuss the nurse's role in assisting the HIV-infected patient with coping, reducing anxiety, minimizing social isolation, and grieving.
- Describe the multidisciplinary approach in caring for a patient with HIV disease.
- List signs and symptoms that might indicate HIV disease.
- List opportunistic infections associated with HIV disease.
- Implement a plan of care for the patient with HIV disease.

KEY TERMS AND DEFINITIONS

_____ 1. Acquired immunodeficiency syndrome (AIDS)
_____ 2. CD4+ lymphocytes
_____ 3. Enzyme-linked immunosorbent assay (ELISA)
_____ 4. HIV infection
_____ 5. Human immunodeficiency virus (HIV)
_____ 6. Kaposi's sarcoma (KS)
_____ 7. Phagocytes
_____ 8. *Pneumocystis carinii* pneumonia (PCP)
_____ 9. Retrovirus
_____ 10. Seroconversion
_____ 11. Seronegative
_____ 12. Surveillance
_____ 13. Vertical transmission
_____ 14. Viral load
_____ 15. Western blot test

a. An unusual pulmonary disease caused by a parasite that is primarily associated with persons who have suppressed immune systems
b. A laboratory blood test to detect the presence of antibodies to a specific antigen, which is a more specific, confirmatory test for HIV
c. The development of detectable levels of antibodies has not occurred, and it would make it impossible to detect HIV in a newly infected person
d. A retrovirus that causes AIDS
e. The best marker when monitoring the immunodeficiency of the HIV disease
f. An antibody test that detects the presence of antibodies to HIV

g. An acquired disease that impairs the body's ability to fight disease; the end stage of HIV infection
h. The transmission of HIV from mother to newborn
i. The exercise of continuous scrutiny of and watchfulness over the distribution and spread of infections and factors related to sufficient accuracy and completeness to be pertinent to effective control
j. White blood cells that are able to surround, engulf, and digest microorganisms and cellular debris
k. A rare cancer of the skin or mucous membranes characterized by blue, red, or purple raised lesions
l. Detectable levels of HIV in the blood
m. A virus composed of genetic material called RNA (ribonucleic acid) instead of the more common DNA (deoxyribonucleic acid) found in most living cells; replicates by converting RNA to DNA
n. The state in which HIV enters the body and multiplies
o. The amount of measurable HIV virions, usually highest immediately after infection and the later stages of the disease

REINFORCING KEY POINTS

1. Explain how HIV disease affects the immune system.

2. Discuss the prevalence of HIV disease in the United States.

3. Name the virus that causes HIV disease.

4. Explain what *retrovirus* means.

5. Discuss the persons at high risk for HIV disease.

6. List the three major routes of transmission of HIV disease.

7. Outline the signs and symptoms the HIV disease patient will exhibit.

8. Describe the lesion of Kaposi's sarcoma.

9. Name the diagnostic tests that are used in HIV disease testing.

APPLICATION OF CLINICAL SKILLS

1. Write a nursing care plan for the HIV disease patient with the emphasis on emotional support.

2. Consider the risks that health care workers take regarding occupational exposure to HIV.

3. Describe the precautions taken when caring for an HIV disease patient.

4. With another student, role play counseling a patient who has just tested positive for HIV.

EXERCISES IN FUNDAMENTAL CONCEPTS

1. The _____ is an agency of the U. S. government that provides facilities and services for the investigation, identification, prevention, and control of disease.

2. _____ is defined as an acquired condition that impairs the body's ability to fight disease; it is the end stage of a continuum of _____.

3. _____ is a broad diagnostic term that includes the pathologic condition and clinical illness caused by HIV infection. It replaces previously used terms, such as AIDS-related complex (ARC) and AIDS.

4. HIV is an *obligate virus*, meaning _____.

5. The three most common modes of HIV transmission are _____, _____, and _____.

6. Seroconversion occurs in 95% of persons within _____ and 99% of persons within _____ of exposure to HIV.

7. Men who have sex with men accounted for only 50% of the total AIDS cases in the United States. _____ and _____ constitute a fast-growing segment of the population with HIV disease.

8. _____ is the development of antibodies to HIV that takes place approximately 5 days to 3 months after exposure, generally within 1 to 3 weeks.

EXERCISES IN CRITICAL THINKING

Topics for Writing
1. Sketch the progression from initial infection with HIV to full-blown HIV disease.

2. Sketch the replication of a retrovirus.

3. List the major prevention options that offer no risk or a reduced risk of contracting HIV.

Topics for Discussion
1. Discuss the trends of the distribution of HIV disease, taking into consideration not only culture, but also age-groups.

2. Describe the major functions of HIV testing and counseling as recommended by the CDC.

3. Discuss ways the nurse can provide emotional support to the person with HIV disease.

STUDY QUESTIONS

1. The retrovirus HIV affects the immune system because it attacks the:
   a. B cells
   b. Platelets
   c. Red blood cells
   d. CD_4 + lymphocytes

2. Mrs. Davis has been told that she is HIV infected. Patient teaching includes the fact that once exposed, symptoms of HIV disease may not become obvious for:
   a. 1 week
   b. 1 to 2 days
   c. 2 to 6 weeks
   d. Up to 10 years

3. The first blood test used to screen for the presence of HIV antibodies is:
   a. ELISA
   b. Western blot
   c. HIV group IV
   d. Electrophoresis

4. The medication regime that presently offers the greatest hope for HIV disease is:
   a. EFT
   b. Zidovudine (AZT)
   c. Acyclovir
   d. Drugs used in combination

5. In patient teaching regarding the prevention of HIV disease, the nurse warns that the fastest-growing segment of the population with HIV disease is:
   a. Bisexual men
   b. Married women
   c. Bisexual women
   d. Women and children

6. What makes the HIV retrovirus different is that it is composed of the genetic material:
   a. DNA
   b. RNA
   c. T cells
   d. B cells

7. Mrs. Brannon fears that she may have been exposed to HIV 8 years ago when she had a blood transfusion. The nurse tells Mrs. Brannon that the person most at risk for contracting HIV through blood transfusions is the patient who was administered blood before:
   a. 1980
   b. 1982
   c. 1985
   d. 1990

8. When the patient is prescribed zidovudine (AZT), important patient teaching includes:
   a. Discontinuing it if vomiting occurs
   b. Having blood counts done every 2 weeks
   c. Getting an abortion if pregnancy occurs
   d. Must be taken exactly as ordered

9. Nutritional recommendations for the HIV disease patient should emphasize:
   a. Low calorie, low fat
   b. Low protein, high fiber
   c. High calorie, low potassium
   d. High calorie, high potassium

10. Mr. Burton states that he has been having night sweats. He states that his lover also has the same problem. He asks the nurse, "What should I do?" The nurse would recommend:
    a. Flu shots
    b. HIV testing
    c. Protected sex
    d. Medications for AIDS

11. A new mother is distressed because she has been told that both she and her new baby are HIV positive. This transmission of HIV from mother to child is called:
    a. Inherited gene
    b. Maternal HIV
    c. Genetic exposure
    d. Vertical transmission

12. Mr. Owens asks to be tested for HIV because his lover was recently diagnosed as HIV positive. He asks the nurse how long he will have to wait before he finds out he is also HIV positive. The nurse replies:
    a. "It usually takes 1 year to know."
    b. "We never know. Each patient is different."
    c. "It depends on the kind of test your doctor orders."
    d. "Antibodies usually are detected within 1 to 3 weeks of exposure."

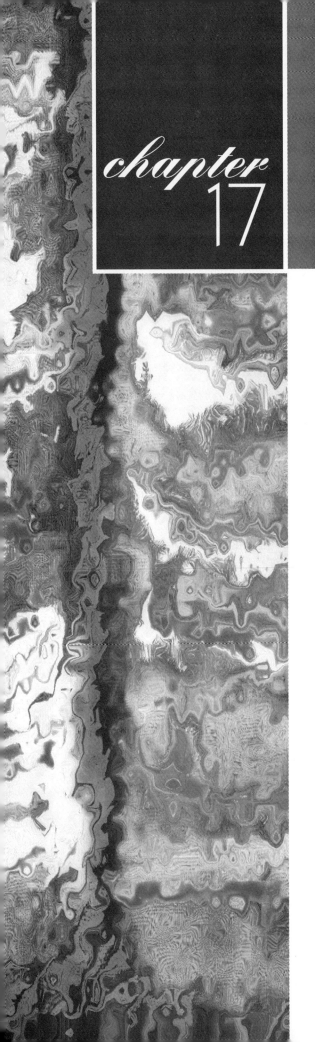

chapter 17

Care of the Patient with Cancer

CHAPTER SUMMARY

Chapter 17 describes the risk factors and seven warning signs of cancer. It defines the terminology used to describe cellular changes, characteristics of malignant cells, and types of malignancies. The diagnostic tests that are specific for cancer are described along with a detailed explanation of tumor classification. Medications used in the treatment of cancer and dramatic symptoms of cancer are discussed. The nursing interventions for cancer patients who undergo surgery, radiation therapy, chemotherapy, immunotherapy, and bone marrow transplantation are explained in detail.

LEARNING OBJECTIVES

After reading the chapter in the textbook and working through the chapter in this study guide, the student should be able to do the following:

- Define the key terms found in the matching exercises.
- List seven risk factors for the development of cancer.
- State seven warning signs of cancer.
- Indicate the incidence of cancer as one of the leading causes of death in the United States.

- Define terminology used to describe cellular changes, characteristics of malignant cells, and types of malignancies.
- Describe the major categories of chemotherapeutic agents.
- Describe the process of metastasis.
- Explain common reasons for delay in seeking medical care when a diagnosis of cancer is suspected.
- List common diagnostic tests used to identify the presence of cancer.
- Explain why biopsy is essential in confirming a diagnosis of cancer.
- Define the systems of tumor classification, that is, grading and staging.
- Discuss six general guidelines for the use of pain relief measures for the patient with advanced cancer.
- Describe the nursing interventions for the individual undergoing surgery, radiation therapy, chemotherapy, or bone marrow transplantation.

KEY TERMS AND DEFINITIONS

_____ 1. Biopsy
_____ 2. Cachexia
_____ 3. Carcinoma
_____ 4. Immunosurveillance
_____ 5. Leukopenia
_____ 6. Malignant
_____ 7. Metastasis
_____ 8. Neoplasm
_____ 9. Palliative
_____ 10. Papanicolaou test
_____ 11. Sarcoma
_____ 12. Stomatitis
_____ 13. Thrombocytopenia

a. Process by which tumor cells spread to distant parts of the body
b. An abnormal hematological condition in which the number of platelets is reduced
c. Abnormal decrease in the number of white blood cells to fewer than 5000/mm^3
d. Ill health, malnutrition, and wasting as a result of chronic disease
e. To soothe or relieve intensity of uncomfortable symptoms but not to produce a cure
f. Cancerous; tumors tending or threatening to cause death
g. Method of examining stained cells obtained from lesions, and other material by aspiration, scraping, a smear, or washing of the tissue; the Pap test is a vital part of the female pelvic examination to detect cancer of the cervix
h. The immune system's recognition and destruction of newly developed abnormal cells
i. A malignant tumor
j. Any inflammatory condition of the mouth; may result from drugs used for cancer
k. Malignant neoplasm of connective tissue arising in fibrous, fatty, muscular, synovial, vascular, or neural tissue
l. Any abnormal growth of new tissue, which may be benign or malignant
m. Removal of a small piece of living tissue for microscopic examination to confirm or establish a diagnosis of cancer

REINFORCING KEY POINTS

1. Define the term *oncology*.

2. Name the kind of cancer that causes the highest number of deaths.

3. Discuss the primary sites where cancer frequently originates.

4. Define the word *carcinogen*, and give an example.

5. Discuss the major risk factors involved in causing cancer.

6. List the foods that are recommended to reduce the risk of cancer.

7. Cite the seven warning signs of cancer.

8. Define neoplasm and carcinoma, and differentiate between the two.

9. Differentiate between a malignant and a benign neoplasm.

10. Describe the meaning of metastasis.

11. Explain what it means for a tumor to be "most differentiated" or "least differentiated."

12. Describe the tumor, node, and metastasis (TNM) staging classification system.

13. Cite the meaning of Pap test results:
   a. Class 1

   b. Class 2

   c. Class 3

   d. Class 4

   e. Class 5

14. Explain why a biopsy is important when cancer is suspected.

15. Identify the four types of biopsies in the figure below:

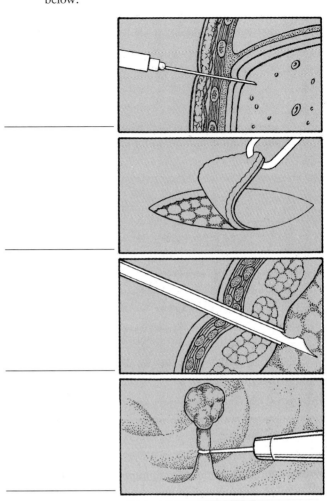

_____

_____

_____

_____

16. Discuss how radiation therapy is used to cure or control cancer.

17. Outline the side effects of chemotherapy that the nurse should be alert for in the patient who is receiving these agents.

APPLICATION OF CLINICAL SKILLS

1. Write a care plan for the patient with internal radiation treatment.

2. Teach a patient the risk factors of cancer and how to avoid those factors.

3. Explain to a woman what a mammogram is and how the results are used to fight cancer.

4. Instruct a woman on how to perform breast self-examination.

5. Explain the meaning of a Pap test when the results are class 2.

6. Instruct a patient on the seven warning signs of cancer and how to assess for each.

7. Explain the purpose of a biopsy.

8. Instruct a man on how to perform a testicular self-examination.

EXERCISES IN FUNDAMENTAL CONCEPTS

1. Cancer is not one disease but a group of diseases characterized by _____ _____.

2. _____ is the term used for various factors that are possible origins of cancer. _____ are substances known to increase the risk for the development of cancer.

3. _____ is the term for uncontrolled or abnormal growth of cells and may be benign (not recurrent or progressive) or malignant (cancerous) resisting treatment.

4. _____ is the process by which tumor cells are spread to distant parts of the body.

5. Immunosurveillance is the immune system's _____.

6. _____ is the term used for malignant tumors composed of epithelial cells with a tendency to metastasize. _____ refers to the malignant tumor of connective tissues, such as muscle or bone.

7. Tumors are classified grade 1 to grade 4 by the degree of malignancy. Grade 1 is the _____ tumor (most like parent tissue) and the _____. Grade 4 is the _____ tumor and most unlike parent tissue; it is highly malignant.

8. The only definite way to determine the presence of malignant cells is to obtain a tissue _____, which is the removal of a small piece of living tissue from an organ or other part of the body.

9. Palliative therapy is designed to _____ but does not produce a _____.

10. _____ is a reduction in the number of circulating white blood cells because of depression of the bone marrow and is a common problem for patients receiving chemotherapy that can lead to life-threatening infections.

11. _____ is a reduction in the number of circulating platelets caused by the depression of the bone marrow.

EXERCISES IN CRITICAL THINKING

Topics for Writing

1. List the six major classifications of medications used in cancer chemotherapy and the common side effects of each.

2. Write a care plan for the cancer patient with gastrointestinal complications.

Topics for Discussion

1. Discuss why certain foods are believed to contribute to causing cancer and why certain others are believed to be preventive.

2. Discuss the different ways that a diagnosis of cancer is made.

3. Consider pain management for the patient in the advanced stages of cancer.

STUDY QUESTIONS

1. Mrs. Bradford, 32 years old, has been diagnosed with breast cancer. She asks the nurse, "What are my chances of being cured?" The nurse states that the most important key in the curing of cancer is:
   a. Radiotherapy
   b. Chemotherapy
   c. Early diagnosis
   d. Location of neoplasm

2. *Neoplasm* is the term referring to:
   a. Benign tumors
   b. Malignant tumors
   c. Metastatic tumors
   d. All tumors, benign or malignant

3. The invasive process of malignant tumors spreading to other parts of the body away from the primary site of the cancer is called:
   a. Neoplasm
   b. Anaplasia
   c. Metastasis
   d. Transformation

4. Mr. Goings, 50 years old, has been diagnosed with a malignant tumor of connective tissue. This is documented as:
   a. Sarcoma
   b. Teratoma
   c. Melanoma
   d. Carcinoma

5. Malignant growths have the following characteristic:
   a. Slow growth
   b. Encapsulated tumor
   c. Well-differentiated cells
   d. Tumor invading normal tissue

6. Ms. Melrose, an oncology nurse, is explaining to Mrs. Dean, who has been diagnosed with pancreatic cancer, the concept of staging and classification of tumors. She tells her that staging refers to classification of tumors according to:
   a. Spread of cancer
   b. Duration of cancer
   c. Characteristics of cells
   d. Recurrence of cancer

7. During a routine self-examination, Mrs. Gibson, 36 years old, finds a lump in her breast. Mrs. Gibson is told that the following test is necessary to establish a diagnosis of breast cancer:
   a. White blood cell count (WBC)
   b. Mammogram
   c. Biopsy of lump
   d. Exploratory surgery

8. When used with a TNM designation, the number indicates:
   a. The degree of malignancy, with no metastasis present
   b. The degree of malignancy, with 4 being the most malignant
   c. The degree of metastasis, with 4 being the most widespread
   d. The degree of malignancy, with 1 being the most malignant

9. The only definitive way to diagnose cancer is with a (an):
   a. Biopsy
   b. Computed tomography (CT) scan
   c. Lumpectomy
   d. X-ray examination

10. Mrs. Davis, 42 years old, is scheduled for external radiation treatments. During the course of this treatment the nurse should be especially alert for the following problem:
    a. Constipation
    b. Ulcers in mouth
    c. Severe immobility
    d. Impaired skin integrity

11. Mr. Smith is upset because his chemotherapy is causing hair loss. He is told that alopecia is common when a patient is receiving chemotherapy. It is important to teach the patient that the loss of hair is:
    a. Rare
    b. Avoidable
    c. Permanent
    d. Not permanent

12. One of the final effects of cancer on the body is:
    a. Cachexia
    b. Metastasis
    c. Loss of smell
    d. Loss of sensation

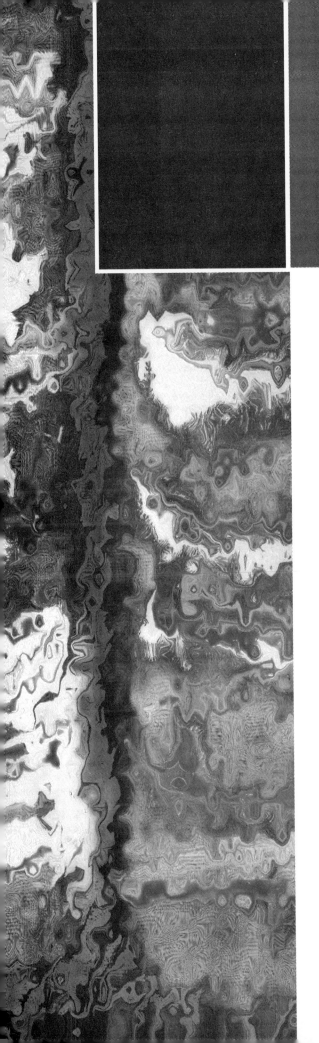

Answer Key

CHAPTER 1

Key Terms and Definitions

1. n
2. l
3. b
4. j
5. r
6. q
7. f
8. h
9. o
10. d
11. p
12. a
13. i
14. e
15. m
16. c
17. k
18. g

Reinforcing Key Points

1. p. 2
2. p. 2
3. p. 2
4. p. 6
5. pp. 6, 7
6. p. 7
7. p. 8
8. p. 10
9. p. 9
10. p. 10
11. p. 11
12. p. 13

Exercises in Fundamental Concepts

1. In anatomical terminology, posterior means toward the back.

2. The term *lateral* means toward the side.

3. The protein factories inside the cell are ribosomes.

4. The substance that contains the genetic code, or blueprint, of the body is DNA.

5. Cell division actually begins to take place during the following stage of mitosis, which is called anaphase.

6. Each body cell in humans contains 46 chromosomes, and chromosomes exist and work in pairs.

7. The study, classification, and description of structures and organs of the body are known as anatomy.

8. The process and function of the body, its structures, and how they interrelate with one another are known as physiology.

9. The tissue that is primarily responsible for the protection of the body is epithelial.

10. The word used to describe a part of the body nearest the origin of the structure or nearest the trunk is proximal.

11. The sagittal plane of the body runs lengthwise from the front to the back.

12. The thoracic cavity contains the heart, blood vessels, and lungs; whereas the abdominal cavity contains the liver, gallbladder, stomach, pancreas, and intestines.

Study Questions

1. c
2. c
3. a
4. b
5. d
6. a
7. d
8. a
9. a

CHAPTER 2

Key Terms and Definitions

1. f
2. d
3. i
4. k
5. l
6. b
7. e
8. n
9. h
10. m
11. a
12. g
13. j
14. c

Reinforcing Key Points

1. p. 18
2. p. 18
3. p. 18
4. p. 18
5. p. 19
6. p. 21
7. p. 19
8. p. 19
9. p. 19
10. pp. 19, 20
11. p. 20
12. p. 20
13. p. 21
14. p. 20
15. p. 21
16. a–c, p. 22
17. p. 22
18. p. 19

Exercises in Fundamental Concepts

1. The word *immune* is derived from the Latin word that means "free from burden."

2. The ability of the immune system to mobilize and use its antibodies and other responses to stimulation by antigen is called immunocompetence.

3. Immunity is the quality of being insusceptible to or unaffected by a particular disease or condition.

4. **Antibodies** develop naturally after infection or **artificially** after vaccinations.

5. Lymphocytes include the T and B cells and the large, granular lymphocytes also known as <u>natural killer cells.</u>

6. <u>T cells</u> are responsible for cell-mediated immunity and provide the body with protection against viruses, fungi, and parasites.

7. An <u>antigen</u> is a substance recognized as foreign that can trigger an immune response.

8. B cells cause the production of antibodies and <u>proliferate</u> (increase in number) in response to a particular antigen.

9. The process by which resistance to an infectious disease is induced or increased is known as <u>immunization.</u>

10. When T cells are activated by an antigen, the process known as <u>cellular immunity</u> occurs.

11. The complement system is activated when an <u>antigen</u> and an <u>antibody</u> interact.

Study Questions

1. d
2. c
3. c
4. d
5. a
6. c
7. b
8. c
9. c
10. b

CHAPTER 3

Key Terms and Definitions

1. h
2. a
3. m
4. d
5. i
6. o
7. n
8. b
9. g

10. l
11. e
12. j
13. c
14. f
15. k

Reinforcing Key Points

1. pp. 33, 45
2. p. 47
3. p. 47
4. p. 48
5. p. 50
6. p. 31
7. p. 32
8. p. 35
9. p. 48
10. pp. 41, 48
11. a-d, p. 31
12. p. 56
13. p. 40
14. p. 57
15. p. 36

Exercises in Fundamental Concepts

1. <u>Surgery</u> is defined as the branch of medicine concerned with disease and trauma requiring an operative procedure.

2. <u>Ablation</u> is an amputation or excision of any part of the body or removal of a growth or harmful substance.

3. <u>Palliative</u> therapy is designed to relieve or reduce intensity of uncomfortable symptoms without cure.

4. <u>Preoperative nursing</u> refers to the role of the nurse during the preoperative, intraoperative, and postoperative phases of a patient's surgical experience.

5. Diabetes increases susceptibility to <u>infection</u> and may <u>impair wound healing</u> from altered glucose metabolism and associated impairment.

6. The patient's bill of rights affirms that the patient must give <u>informed consent</u> (permission obtained from a patient to perform a specific test or procedure) before the beginning of any procedure.

Study Questions

1. d
2. c
3. a
4. b
5. b
6. c
7. d
8. b
9. c
10. b
11. a
12. b
13. c

CHAPTER 4

Key Terms and Definitions

1. f
2. b
3. j
4. d
5. h
6. a
7. g
8. c
9. i
10. e

Reinforcing Key Points

1. p. 61
2. pp. 61, 62
3. a-h, p. 67
4. pp. 68, 69
5. p. 70
6. p. 70
7. pp. 73–75
8. p. 76
9. p. 77
10. p. 88
11. p. 90
12. p. 92

Exercises in Fundamental Concepts

1. The integument is really the body's protector—its first line of defense against infection and injury. In addition to protection, its main function is homeostasis.

2. The skin functions in the prevention and loss of body fluids and in the regulation of body temperature.

3. The inner layer of the epidermis receives its blood supply and nutrition from the underlying dermis through the process of diffusion.

4. Melanin is a black or dark brown pigment that occurs naturally in the hair, skin, and iris and choroid of the eye and is responsible for skin color. Skin color is inherited.

5. When the patient has a skin disorder a way to assess the chief complaint is PQRST, which stands for provocative/palliative, quality/-quantity, region, severity, and time.

6. Hypoxemia is decreased oxygen and is indicated by clubbing of the fingertips.

7. Herpes zoster is caused by the chickenpox virus and is commonly known as shingles.

Study Questions

1. d
2. a
3. d
4. b
5. c
6. c
7. b
8. c
9. b
10. d
11. a
12. a
13. a
14. a
15. b
16. c
17. a
18. a
19. c
20. c

CHAPTER 5

Key Terms and Definitions

1. m
2. d
3. n
4. c
5. l
6. g
7. b
8. h
9. a
10. k
11. f
12. e
13. j
14. i

Reinforcing Key Points

1. p. 103
2. p. 104
3. p. 107
4. p. 107
5. p. 112
6. p. 112
7. p. 112
8. p. 112
9. p. 115
10. pp. 117, 120
11. p. 122
12. p. 129
13. a-g, p. 133
14. p. 147
15. pp. 151, 152
16. p. 153
17. p. 154
18. p. 154
19. p. 158
20. pp. 162, 163
21. p. 133

Exercises in Fundamental Concepts

1. The skeletal system has five basic functions: support, protection, movement, mineral storage, and hemopoiesis.

2. Hemopoiesis is blood cell formation and takes place in the red bone marrow.

3. There are four classifications of the bones, based on their form and shape: long, short, flat, and irregular.

4. Muscle tissue is under voluntary or involuntary control. Voluntary muscle is under conscious control, whereas involuntary muscle tissue responds to internal commands without any conscious control of it.

5. Muscle cells, in union with the nerve cells that control them, are called a motor unit.

6. The impulse from the nerve cell must travel across a small gap, since the nerve cell and the muscle cell do not directly touch each other. This small gap is called a synaptic cleft.

7. A special chemical that travels through the fluid to stimulate the muscle fiber is called a neurotransmitter.

8. Acetylcholine is the specific neurotransmitter for the skeletal muscle tissue.

9. Muscle cells are governed by the "all or nothing" law, which states that when a muscle cell is adequately stimulated or shocked, it will contract completely.

10. Skeletal muscles are usually classified into two broad categories: axial and appendicular.

11. The axial muscle groups are those muscles located on the head, face, neck, and trunk.

12. The appendicular muscle groups are all the muscles of the extremities.

13. The musculoskeletal system provides protection, support, and movement for the body.

14. Circulatory status is assessed by signs of coolness, pallor, cyanosis, and pulse.

15. A test of the rate of capillary refill, which signals circulation status, is called capillary nail refill test.

16. A circulation check is also known as a neurovascular assessment and includes assessment of circulation, motion, and sensation.

17. Remember the 5 P's when conducting a neurovascular assessment:
    a. Pulselessness
    b. Paresthesia (numbness or tingling sensation)
    c. Pallor
    d. Puffiness (edema)
    e. Pain

Study Questions

1. c
2. d
3. a
4. d
5. b
6. c
7. c
8. d
9. d
10. d
11. b
12. d
13. d
14. d
15. d
16. d
17. d
18. d
19. c
20. b
21. d
22. b
23. c
24. b
25. a
26. d
27. b

CHAPTER 6

Key Terms and Definitions

1. f
2. k
3. c
4. i
5. l
6. b
7. h
8. d
9. j
10. e
11. g
12. a

Reinforcing Key Points

1. p. 169
2. p. 168
3. p. 173
4. p. 173
5. pp. 173, 174
6. p. 176
7. p. 177
8. p. 181
9. p. 182
10. p. 183
11. p. 186
12. p. 188
13. p. 190
14. a, p. 196; b, p. 193; c, p. 191
15. p. 198
16. pp. 206, 207
17. p. 208
18. p. 209
19. p. 175

Exercises in Fundamental Concepts

1. Alimentary canal is a musculomembranous tube extending from the mouth to the anus and is approximately 30 feet long.

2. The entrance to the stomach is the cardiac sphincter (so named because of its proximity to the heart); the exit is the pyloric sphincter.

3. The inner surface of the small intestine contains millions of tiny, fingerlike projections clustered over the entire mucous surface called villi.

4. The liver is the largest glandular organ in the body and one of the most complex. It is located just inferior to the diaphragm, covering most of the upper right and extending into the left epigastrium.

5. The hypothalamus contains two centers that affect eating. One center stimulates the individual to eat, and the other signals the individual to stop eating.

6. The Bernstein test is an acid-perfusion test that is used to reproduce the symptoms of gastroesophageal reflux. It aids in differentiating esophageal pain caused by esophageal reflux from that caused by angina pectoris.

7. Candida is a fungal organism normally present in the mucous membrane of the mouth, intestinal tract, and vagina. Candidiasis appears as small white patches on the mucous membranes of the mouth and the tongue.

8. Kaposi's sarcoma is a malignant skin tumor that is seen with increased frequency as a nonsquamous tumor of the oral cavity in patients with AIDS. These lesions are purple and nonulcerated.

Study Questions

1. c
2. b
3. b
4. b
5. d
6. b
7. c
8. b
9. b
10. d
11. b
12. b
13. b
14. d
15. c

CHAPTER 7

Key Terms and Definitions

1. b
2. a
3. f
4. i
5. c
6. k
7. g
8. e
9. j
10. h
11. d

Reinforcing Key Points

1. p. 215
2. p. 217
3. p. 219
4. p. 223
5. p. 224
6. p. 229

Exercises in Fundamental Concepts

1. Although elevation of serum enzymes is found in pathological liver conditions, the tests are not specific for liver disease alone.

2. One way to assess the functional status of the liver is to measure the albumin.

3. Ascites is the accumulation of fluid and albumin in the peritoneal cavity.

4. Paracentesis is a procedure in which fluid is withdrawn from the abdominal cavity that will relieve ascites and also provide fluid for laboratory examination.

5. Hepatitis is an inflammation of the liver resulting from several causes, including viral agents, bacterial agents, or exposure to toxic substances.

Study Questions

1. d
2. c
3. d
4. d
5. b
6. b
7. c
8. a
9. b
10. c
11. d
12. b

CHAPTER 8

Key Terms and Definitions

1. m
2. e
3. o
4. g
5. p
6. b
7. j
8. l
9. c
10. n
11. i
12. a
13. f

14. k
15. d
16. h

Reinforcing Key Points

1. p. 247
2. p. 245
3. p. 247
4. p. 248
5. p. 251
6. pp. 248, 259, 264
7. p. 270
8. pp. 248, 265, 272
9. p. 272
10. p. 289
11. pp. 289, 293
12. p. 285

Exercises in Fundamental Concepts

1. The main function of the cardiovascular system is that it delivers <u>oxygen</u> and <u>nutrients</u> to the cells.

2. The upper right chamber, the <u>right atrium</u>, receives deoxygenated blood from the entire body.

3. The heart has two atrioventricular (AV) valves. They are located between the <u>atrium</u> and <u>ventricle</u>.

4. The left AV valve is composed of cusps (bicuspid) and is commonly called the <u>mitral valve</u>. It is located between the <u>left atrium</u> and <u>ventricle</u>.

5. The heartbeat is initiated in the <u>sinoatrial (SA) node</u>, which is located in the upper part of the right atrium. Because it regulates the beat of the heart, it is known as the <u>pacemaker</u>.

6. The cardiac cycle refers to a <u>complete heartbeat</u>.

7. The phase of contraction is called <u>systole</u>, and the phase of relaxation is called <u>diastole</u>.

8. There are three main types of blood vessels organized to carry blood to and from the heart: capillaries connect the <u>arteries</u> to the <u>veins</u>.

Study Questions

1. d
2. d
3. d

4. c
5. b
6. c
7. c
8. a
9. d
10. c
11. b
12. c
13. c
14. c
15. c
16. d
17. b
18. c
19. d
20. d
21. c
22. c
23. c
24. d

CHAPTER 9

Key Terms and Definitions

1. e
2. b
3. g
4. j
5. i
6. f
7. l
8. a
9. c
10. h
11. k
12. d

Reinforcing Key Points

1. pp. 302–304
2. p. 302
3. p. 302
4. a, p. 305; b, p. 302; c, p. 303
5. p. 305
6. p. 305
7. p. 316
8. a, p. 314; b, p. 313; c, p. 317; d, p. 316

Exercises in Fundamental Concepts

1. Blood is a viscous (thick), red fluid that contains <u>red blood cells</u>, <u>white blood cells</u>, and <u>platelets</u>, which are suspended in a light yellow fluid called <u>plasma</u>.

2. Blood is slightly <u>alkaline</u>, with a pH range of 7.35 to 7.45.

3. The blood performs three critical functions. First, it <u>transports oxygen</u> and <u>nutrition</u> to the cell and waste products away from the cells. Second, it <u>regulates the acid-base balance (pH)</u> with buffers, aids with body temperature because of its water content, and controls the water content as a result of dissolved sodium ions. Third, it <u>protects the body against infection</u> with special cells and prevents blood loss with special clotting mechanisms.

4. <u>Red blood cells (RBCs)</u> give blood its rich color.

5. The average life span of an RBC is <u>120 days</u>.

6. WBCs are called <u>leukocytes</u> and respond predictably to symptoms of infection.

7. A differential white blood cell count is <u>an examination in which the different kinds of WBCs are counted and reported as percentages of the total examined</u>.

8. Platelets are called <u>thrombocytes</u> and function in the <u>prevention of blood loss</u>.

9. A person's blood group or type is determined <u>genetically</u> and <u>inherited from parents</u>.

10. <u>Type O blood</u> can be used in an emergency as donor blood without the danger of anti-A or anti-B antibodies clumping its RBCs and is called universal donor blood.

11. <u>Blood type AB</u> has been called the universal recipient blood because it contains neither anti-A nor anti-B antibodies in its plasma.

Study Questions

1. d
2. c
3. c
4. a
5. b
6. d
7. b
8. d
9. d
10. b
11. c
12. c

CHAPTER 10

Key Terms and Definitions

1. b
2. i
3. c
4. g
5. d
6. k
7. a
8. h
9. f
10. l
11. j
12. e

Reinforcing Key Points

1. p. 338
2. p. 339
3. pp. 339, 341
4. p. 341
5. p. 341
6. p. 342
7. p. 343
8. p. 344
9. p. 344
10. p. 345
11. p. 346
12. p. 346–348
13. a, p. 347; b, p. 347; c, p. 347; d, p. 347
14. p. 353
15. a-d, p. 348
16. p. 349
17. pp. 349, 350
18. pp. 351, 352
19. p. 352
20. a, p. 354; b, p. 354; c, p. 355; d, p. 357; e, p. 355; f, p. 353
21. p. 356
22. p. 360
23. p. 361
24. p. 361
25. p. 365
26. p. 367
27. p. 373
28. p. 340

Exercises in Fundamental Concepts

1. The urinary system is probably the most important system in <u>maintaining homeostasis.</u>

2. Because of the size and shape of the liver, the <u>right</u> kidney lies slightly lower than the left.

3. The <u>nephron</u> is the functional unit of the kidney, and each kidney contains more than <u>1 million</u> nephrons. Its function is to <u>filter the blood</u> and <u>process the urine.</u>

4. <u>Blood pressure</u>, or hydrostatic pressure, determines the glomerular filtration rate (GFR).

5. The body forms <u>1000</u> to <u>2000 ml</u> of urine per day.

6. Urine is <u>slightly acidic</u> with a pH of <u>4.6</u> to <u>8.0.</u>

7. When the bladder contains approximately <u>250 ml</u> of urine, the individual has a conscious desire to urinate.

8. A moderately full bladder holds <u>450 ml</u> (1 pint) of urine.

Study Questions

1. c
2. b
3. a
4. b
5. c
6. b
7. c
8. b
9. c
10. b
11. b
12. b
13. c
14. c
15. c
16. b
17. a

CHAPTER 11

Key Terms and Definitions

1. i
2. f
3. k
4. d
5. m
6. g
7. j
8. c
9. p
10. h
11. n
12. b
13. o
14. q
15. l
16. a
17. e

Reinforcing Key Points

1. pp. 385–387
2. p. 386
3. pp. 386, 411
4. p. 387
5. p. 387
6. p. 388
7. p. 388
8. a, p. 388; b, p. 390; c, p. 390; d, p. 390; e, p. 389; f, p. 390; g, p. 390; h, p. 391; i, p. 391; j, p. 390
9. a, p. 392; b, p. 394; c, p. 395
10. p. 396
11. p. 397
12. p. 397

Exercises in Fundamental Concepts

1. The pharynx, or <u>throat</u>, is the passageway for both <u>air</u> and <u>water.</u>

2. Because the inner lining of the <u>pharynx</u> and the <u>eustachian tube</u> are continuous, an infection of the pharynx can spread easily to the ear.

3. <u>Cilia</u> are small, hairlike processes on the outer surfaces of small cells, aiding metabolism by producing motion or current in a fluid.

4. When a patient has a tracheostomy he or she cannot speak because <u>breathing occurs through one tracheal opening, so that air cannot pass over the vocal cords, making speech physiologically impossible.</u>

5. When a foreign object is aspirated, it is most likely to enter the <u>right bronchus.</u>

6. Gas exchange of <u>air</u> and <u>carbon dioxide</u> by the process of <u>diffusion</u> takes place in a single grapelike structure called an <u>alveolus.</u>

7. The normal range of respirations for an adult is 16 to 32 respirations/min.

8. Specialized receptors that are sensitive to carbon dioxide and oxygen levels in the blood and can modify respiratory rates are called chemoreceptors.

9. Carbon dioxide is the chemical stimulant for the regulation of respirations. Therefore, when the blood becomes acidic, respirations increase.

10. Difficulty breathing, or dyspnea, is a subjective experience that the patient describes.

11. Orthopnea is an abnormal condition in which a person must sit or stand in order to breathe deeply or comfortably.

12. The presence of adventitious sounds indicates abnormal breath sounds.

13. Identify the following breath sounds:
    a. Musical, high-pitched sibilant wheezes
    b. Low-pitched, loud, coarse sonorous wheezes
    c. Short, discrete, bubbling crackles
    d. Low-pitched, grating pleural friction rub

14. The illustration below shows a complete collapse of the right lung called a pneumothorax.

Study Questions

1. d
2. d
3. c
4. a
5. d
6. d
7. d
8. d
9. b
10. c
11. a
12. a
13. d
14. c

CHAPTER 12

Key Terms and Definitions

1. g
2. k
3. e
4. l
5. j
6. d
7. f
8. c
9. i
10. a
11. h
12. b

Reinforcing Key Points

1. p. 436
2. p. 436
3. p. 437
4. p. 436
5. a-f, pp. 436–440;
6. p. 437
7. p. 437
8. p. 439
9. p. 439
10. p. 440
11. p. 443
12. p. 447
13. p. 456
14. p. 457
15. a-e, pp. 459–474
16. p. 461
17. p. 461
18. p. 465
19. p. 436

Exercises in Fundamental Concepts

1. The two broad categories of glands are exocrine and endocrine. Exocrine glands secrete through a series of ducts, such as sebaceous and sudoriferous glands of the skin. Their secretions are protective and functional. Endocrine glands are ductless; they release their secretions directly into the blood stream. Their secretions have a regulatory function.

2. Hormones are chemical messengers that travel through the blood stream to their target organ.

3. The amount of hormonal release is controlled by a negative feedback system, which is a decrease in function in response to stimuli.

4. The pituitary gland is called the master gland because through the negative feedback system it exerts its control over the other endocrine glands.

5. ADH causes the kidneys to conserve water by decreasing the amount of urine produced. ADH is sometimes called vasopressin because it causes constriction of the arterioles in the body, which results in increased blood pressure.

6. Adequate intake of iodine is necessary for the formation of thyroid hormones.

7. When calcium levels are low, the nerve cells become excited and stimulate the muscles with many impulses, resulting in tetany.

8. The two hormones that are released during times of stress are epinephrine or adrenalin and norepinephrine. They can cause the heart rate and blood pressure to increase, the blood vessels to contract, and the liver to release glucose reserves for immediate energy. This is a systemic preparation of the body for the "fight or flight" response that is needed in times of crisis.

9. The islets of Langerhans of the pancreas secrete two major hormones: insulin and glucagon.

10. The two hormones that the ovaries produce are estrogen and progesterone. These hormones are responsible for development of secondary sex characteristics and preparation of the reproductive organs.

11. The testes release the hormone testosterone, which is responsible for the development of the male secondary sex characteristics.

12. The thymus gland plays an active role in the immune system.

13. The pineal gland secretes the hormone melatonin, which is thought to induce sleep and may also affect one's mood.

Study Questions

1. a
2. c
3. a
4. d
5. d
6. b
7. c
8. c
9. c
10. a
11. d
12. b

13. c
14. b
15. b
16. d
17. d
18. b
19. a
20. a
21. d
22. d
23. a
24. c
25. c
26. c
27. a
28. d
29. a

CHAPTER 13

Key Terms and Definitions

1. j
2. d
3. p
4. m
5. g
6. h
7. c
8. e
9. k
10. i
11. f
12. n
13. a
14. b
15. o
16. l

Reinforcing Key Points

1. p. 479
2. p. 479
3. pp. 480, 482
4. p. 483
5. p. 485
6. a, p. 492; b, p. 494; c, p. 494; d, p. 493
7. p. 483
8. pp. 489–491
9. p. 497
10. p. 497
11. p. 499
12. a, p. 502; b, p. 503; c, p. 502; d, p. 504; e, p. 503
13. p. 504

14. p. 505
15. p. 507
16. p. 513
17. p. 515
18. p. 520
19. a, p. 525; b, p. 524; c, p. 525; d, p. 526; e, p. 525
20. a, p. 529; b, p. 529; c, p. 531; d, p. 530; e, p. 528; f, p. 531

Exercises in Fundamental Concepts

1. The testes also produce testosterone, which is responsible for the development of male secondary sex characteristics.

2. Mature sperm, once deposited in the female reproductive system, live approximately 48 hours.

3. During the menstrual cycle, an ovum matures and is released about 14 days before the next menstrual flow. This, on average, occurs every 28 days.

4. Sexuality is often described as the sense of being female or male.

5. Sex usually describes the biological aspects of sexuality, such as genital sexual activity.

6. Gender identity is the sense of being feminine or masculine. Gender role is the manner in which a person acts as female or male.

7. Painful menstruation is called dysmenorrhea, whereas excessive flow is called menorrhagia.

8. Biopsies are procedures in which samples of tissues are taken for evaluation to confirm or locate a lesion.

9. Conization of the cervix is indicated when eroded or infected tissue is to be removed or there is a need for confirmation of cervical cancer.

10. All pregnancy tests, regardless of the method, are based on detection of human chorionic gonadotropin (HCG), which is secreted in the urine after fertilization of the ovum.

11. The climacteric is the phase of the aging process of women and men who are making a transition from a reproductive phase to a nonreproductive phase of life. The female climacteric is called menopause.

12. Endometriosis is a condition in which endometrial tissue appears outside the uterus.

13. Dyspareunia is sexual intercourse accompanied by pain.

14. A fistula is defined as an abnormal opening between two organs and is named for the organs involved.

15. Urethrovaginal fistula is an opening between the urethra and vagina.

16. Vesicovaginal fistula is an opening between the bladder and vagina.

17. Rectovaginal fistula is an opening between the rectum and vagina.

18. A hysterectomy involves the removal of the uterus, including the cervix. A total abdominal hysterectomy with bilateral salpingoooophorectomy (TAH-BSO) is the removal of the uterus, fallopian tubes, and ovaries.

19. Carcinoma in situ is a preinvasive, asymptomatic carcinoma that can only be diagnosed by microscopic examination of cervical cells.

Study Questions

1. b
2. b
3. d
4. c
5. a
6. a
7. b
8. c
9. b
10. c
11. a
12. d
13. c
14. b
15. a
16. d
17. b

CHAPTER 14

Key Terms and Definitions
1. a
2. m
3. h
4. p
5. e
6. n
7. i
8. b
9. l
10. k
11. o
12. f
13. c
14. j
15. d
16. g

Reinforcing Key Points
1. p. 541
2. p. 541
3. a-f, p. 542
4. p. 542
5. p. 543
6. p. 544
7. a, p. 550; b, p. 550; c, p. 550; d, p. 547; e, p. 550; f, p. 546
8. p. 553
9. p. 555
10. p. 556
11. p. 559
12. p. 561
13. a, p. 562; b, p. 565; c, p. 565; d, p. 565
14. p. 569
15. p. 571
16. p. 572
17. p. 577

Exercises in Fundamental Concepts
1. The accessory structures of the eye—the eyebrows, eyelashes, eyelids, and lacrimal apparatus—function mainly as protective devices.

2. The conjunctiva is a thin mucous membrane that lines the inner aspect of the eyelids and the anterior surface of the eyeball to the edge of the cornea.

3. The outermost layer of the eyeball is the fibrous tunic, composed of thick, white, opaque, connective tissue called the sclera, or white of the eye.

4. Intraocular pressure is the pressure within the eyeball.

5. A circular opening in the iris of the eye, located slightly to the nasal side of the center of the iris, is the pupil.

6. The retina is a 10-layered, delicate, nervous tissue membrane of the eye that receives images of external objects and transmits impulses through the optic nerve to the brain.

7. Refraction is the bending of light rays as they pass through the colorless structures of the eye, allowing light from the environment to focus on the retina.

8. Accommodation is the adjustment of the eye for various distances; thus it is able to focus the image of an object on the retina by changing the curvature of the lens.

9. Convergence is the movement of both eyes medially to allow light rays from an object to hit the same point on both retinas.

10. The eustachian canal is lined with mucous membrane that joins the nasopharynx and the middle ear cavity. It is also called the auditory canal.

11. Proprioceptors are any sensory nerve endings, such as those located in muscles, tendons, and joints, that respond to stimuli originating from within the body regarding movement and spatial position; they work in conjunction with the semicircular canals and vestibule of the inner ear to maintain proper coordination.

12. Exophthalmos is an abnormal condition characterized by a marked protrusion of the eyeballs.

Study Questions
1. d
2. c
3. c
4. c
5. d
6. d
7. b
8. d
9. d
10. b
11. b
12. c

13. c
14. d
15. b
16. b
17. b
18. c
19. c

CHAPTER 15

Key Terms and Definitions

1. l
2. g
3. b
4. e
5. j
6. h
7. f
8. a
9. k
10. c
11. i
12. d

Reinforcing Key Points

1. pp. 585–588
2. p. 587
3. p. 588
4. p. 585
5. p. 586
6. p. 588
7. a-d, p. 588
8. p. 586
9. p. 587
10. pp. 585–587
11. a, p. 586; b, p. 585; c, p. 586; d, p. 586; e, p. 586;
    f, p. 586; g, p. 587
12. pp. 587, 588
13. p. 589
14. p. 591
15. p. 594
16. p. 594
17. a, p. 595; b, p. 594; c, p. 596; d, p. 594
18. p. 596
19. p. 597
20. p. 599
21. p. 599
22. p. 600
23. a-d, p. 607
24. p. 609
25. p. 610
26. p. 611

27. p. 614
28. p. 618
29. p. 624
30. p. 625

Exercises in Fundamental Concepts

1. The first division, the central nervous system (CNS), is composed of the brain and the spinal cord.

2. The second component is the peripheral nervous system, which lies outside the central nervous system (CNS).

3. The autonomic system is sometimes called the involuntary nervous system because its action takes place without conscious control.

4. There are 31 pairs of spinal nerves and 12 pairs of cranial nerves.

5. The primary function of the autonomic nervous system is to maintain internal homeostasis; for example, it strives to maintain a normal heartbeat, a constant body temperature, and a normal respiratory pattern.

6. The autonomic system has two divisions: the sympathetic nervous system and the parasympathetic nervous system.

7. A decreasing level of consciousness is the earliest sign of increased intracranial pressure.

8. The Glasgow Coma Scale consists of testing of three parts of the neurological assessment: eye opening, best motor response, and best verbal response.

9. A loss of function is called paralysis; a lesser degree of movement deficit is called paresis.

10. A pupil that is fixed and dilated is sometimes called a blown pupil and is an ominous sign that must be reported to the physician immediately.

11. A widened pulse pressure, increased systolic blood pressure, and bradycardia are together called Cushing's response.

12. Hemiplegia is paralysis of one side of the body.

13. Agnosia is a total or partial loss of the ability to recognize familiar objects or persons through sensory stimuli as a result of organic brain damage.

14. Aura is defined as a sensation, as of light or warmth, that may precede an attack of migraine or an epileptic seizure.

15. Nystagmus is an involuntary, rhythmic movement of the eye; the oscillation may be horizontal, vertical, rotary, or mixed.

16. Bradykinesia is an abnormal condition characterized by slowness of voluntary movements and speech and is present with rigidity and loss of postural reflexes.

17. Apraxia is impairment in the ability to perform purposeful acts and interferes with the ability to carry out daily functions.

18. When a patient fails to recognize that he or she has a paralyzed side, it is called unilateral neglect.

19. Quadriplegics are patients who sustain injuries to one of the cervical segments of the spinal cord. Paraplegics are those whose lesions are confined to the thoracic, lumbar, or sacral segments of the spinal cord.

20. Hyperreflexia is a neurological condition characterized by increased reflex actions.

21. Autonomic dysreflexia occurs as a result of abnormal cardiovascular response to stimulation of the sympathetic division of the autonomic nervous system as a result of stimulation of the bladder, large intestine, or other visceral organs.

Study Questions

1. a
2. b
3. b
4. d
5. a
6. c
7. d
8. d
9. a
10. a
11. c
12. c
13. a

14. b
15. c
16. c
17. b
18. c
19. c
20. a
21. a
22. c
23. c
24. c
25. a
26. a

CHAPTER 16

Key Terms and Definitions

1. g
2. e
3. f
4. n
5. d
6. k
7. j
8. a
9. m
10. l
11. c
12. i
13. h
14. o
15. b

Reinforcing Key Points

1. p. 636
2. p. 637
3. p. 636
4. p. 636
5. p. 637
6. p. 638
7. p. 642
8. p. 636
9. p. 643

Exercises in Fundamental Concepts

1. The Centers for Disease Control and Prevention is an agency of the U.S. government that provides facilities and services for the investigation, identification, prevention, and control of disease.

2. Acquired immunodeficiency syndrome (AIDS) is defined as an acquired condition that impairs the body's ability to fight disease; it is the end stage of a continuum of HIV infection.

3. HIV disease is a broad diagnostic term that includes the pathologic condition and clinical illness caused by HIV infection. It replaces previously used terms, such as AIDS-related complex (ARC) and AIDS.

4. HIV is an *obligate virus*, meaning it must have a host organism to survive.

5. The three most common modes of HIV transmission are anal or vaginal intercourse, contaminated injecting drug equipment/paraphernalia, and from mother to child.

6. Seroconversion occurs in 95% of persons within 3 months and 99% of persons within 6 months of exposure to HIV.

7. Men who have sex with men accounted for only 50% of the total AIDS cases in the United States. Women and children constitute a fast-growing segment of the population with AIDS.

8. Seroconversion is the development of antibodies to HIV that takes place approximately 5 days to 3 months after exposure, generally within 1 to 3 weeks.

Study Questions

1. d
2. d
3. a
4. d
5. b
6. b
7. c
8. d
9. d
10. b
11. d
12. d

CHAPTER 17

Key Terms and Definitions

1. m
2. d
3. i
4. h
5. c
6. f
7. a
8. l
9. e
10. g
11. k
12. j
13. b

Reinforcing Key Points

1. p. 669
2. p. 669
3. p. 669
4. p. 670
5. p. 670
6. p. 670
7. p. 670
8. p. 671
9. p. 671
10. p. 672
11. p. 672
12. p. 672
13. a-e, p. 673
14. p. 673
15. p. 673
16. p. 676
17. p. 676

Exercises in Fundamental Concepts

1. Cancer is not one disease but a group of diseases characterized by uncontrolled growth and spread of abnormal cells.

2. Carcinogenesis is the term used for various factors that are possible origins of cancer. Carcinogens are substances known to increase the risk for the development of cancer.

3. Neoplasm is the term for uncontrolled or abnormal growth of cells and may be benign (not recurrent or progressive) or malignant (cancerous) resisting treatment.

4. Metastasis is the process by which tumor cells are spread to distant parts of the body.

5. Immunosurveillance is the immune system's recognition and destruction of newly developed abnormal cells.

6. Carcinoma is the term used for malignant tumors composed of epithelial cells, with a tendency to metastasize. Sarcoma refers to the malignant tumor of connective tissues, such as muscle or bone.

7. Tumors are classified grade 1 to grade 4 by the degree of malignancy. Grade 1 is the most differentiated tumor (most like parent tissue) and the least malignant. Grade 4 is the least differentiated tumor and most unlike parent tissue; it is highly malignant.

8. The only definite way to determine the presence of malignant cells is to obtain a tissue biopsy, which is the removal of a small piece of living tissue from an organ or other part of the body.

9. Palliative therapy is designed to relieve intensity of painful symptoms but does not produce a cure.

10. Leukopenia is the reduction in the number of circulating white blood cells because of depression of the bone marrow and is a common problem for patients receiving chemotherapy that can lead to life-threatening infections.

11. Thrombocytopenia is a reduction in the number of circulating platelets caused by the depression of the bone marrow.

Study Questions

1. c
2. d
3. c
4. a
5. d
6. a
7. c
8. b
9. a
10. d
11. d
12. a